DIABETIC MEAL PR

Healty & Delicious Meals to Cook, Prep, Grab, and Go - Diabetic Cookbook to Prevent and Reverse Diabetes with 30-Day Meal Plan + Special Desserts

TABLE OF CONTENTS

UNDERSTANDING DIABETES

Diabetes is an intense interminable condition endured by a large number of individuals around the world.

If you have diabetes and neglect to control your blood glucose levels, you are probably going to wind up with at least one genuine ailment, for example, coronary illness, kidney failure, and damaged nerves, among numerous others.

Pre-diabetes is a condition where your blood glucose levels are higher than they ought to be; nevertheless, not all that high that you are recognized as being diabetic. Research suggests that up to 70% of people with pre-diabetes proceed to develop full type 2 diabetes.

In any case, this implies that 30% figure out how to end the advancement of diabetes before it turns into a persistent illness. Thus, if you have been confirmed as pre-diabetic, developing all out diabetes isn't inescapable.

You can't change your past conduct, your age, or your qualities, yet you can change your lifestyle how you disport yourself and what you eat and drink.

HOW YOUR STOMACH
RELATED SYSTEM FUNCTIONS

The foods you eat are, for the most part, a mix of starches, proteins, and fats in different extents. A bit of meat, for instance, contains, for the most part, protein and fats. Vegetables, for example, potatoes contain bunches of sugars.

When you digest a piece of food, it is separated into its key segments, carbs, proteins, and fats. These parts are then separated further in your stomach related system and are passed into your circulation system, which conveys them around your body.

Your energy originates from glucose. Glucose is only a primary sugar. Yet, it is your body's essential wellspring of vitality.

Most glucose originates from processing the sugar and starch in starches that you get from food, for example, rice, pasta, grains, pieces of bread, potatoes, products of the soil vegetables. The glucose created by processing in your stomach is then passed into your circulatory system, which conveys it to your body's cells.

Glucose is the fuel for your cells; it controls your developments, contemplations, and everything else you do.

To control your cells, glucose needs to get into them. It does this with the assistance of insulin.

Insulin is a hormone produced in the body It is delivered by your pancreas. The pancreas discharges insulin into your circulation system, where it goes around your body and gets together with glucose on a similar journey. The motivation behind insulin is to empower glucose to enter your cells.

To do this, insulin connects itself to a receptor in the outside of the cell. This causes the cell layer to permit glucose to enter the cell. The cell would then be able to use glucose as its fuel.

This glucose-insulin system needs to work appropriately if you are to be in control of blood sugar levels.

If the insulin doesn't carry out its function of 'opening the cell entryway' for glucose, the glucose won't have the option to get into the cell... what's more, the cell will come up short on fuel.

Diabetes is a condition where the glucose-insulin system doesn't work effectively.

There are two significant types of diabetes: *(a) type 1 and (b) type 2.* Over 90% of people with diabetes have type 2 diabetes.

In **type 1 diabetes,** the pancreas doesn't create any insulin or best case scenario, practically nothing. Type 1 can't be relieved. The primary way these people with diabetes can cope is by injections of insulin.

In **type 2 diabetes,** the pancreas produces insulin, which is discharged into the circulatory system. When the insulin shows up at a cell, it has trouble appending itself to a receptor. So, it can't incite the cell layer to open and permit glucose to enter the cell.

Insulin opposition is the condition where insulin can't connect itself to cell receptors.

Envision a key attempting to slide into a lock-in an entryway. The key can't get in if the lock is in a stuck state with a piece of chewing gum. There is nothing amiss with the key and nothing amiss with the lock. In any case, before the key can get in, the lock must be cleaned out.

One of the fundamental reasons for insulin opposition is having cell 'entryways' stuck with fat. The best way to 'unjam' them is to wipe out all fat beyond what many would consider possible from your diet for four weeks to about a month and a half (at any rate) until the cell receptors are liberated from fat.

So what do you need to do to prevent type 2 diabetes coming from pre-diabetes to the out and out incessant condition with its raised dangers of respiratory failures, strokes, visual deficiency, kidney transplants, leg removals, and other deplorable conditions?

CHANGE YOUR LIFESTYLE USING

HERE ARE 12 THINGS YOU CAN DO:

1) Avoid Stationary Conduct

A stationary lifestyle is one in which you sit a large portion of the day and embrace minimal physical activity. The connection between inactive conduct and the danger of diabetes is simply demonstrated.

An investigation of the consequences of 47 examinations found that individuals who went through the more significant part of the day occupied with inactive conduct (e.g., office laborers) have a 91% danger of creating diabetes.

If you work in an office, there are a few different ways you can change your inactive propensities:

- Stand up from your work area and stroll around for a couple of moments consistently.

- Stand as opposed to sitting when chatting on the telephone.

- Take the steps rather than the lift.

- Park far away from the grocery store, so you need to walk a decent separation to get inside.

- Go for long strolls at night (simple if you have a pooch).

- The ideal approach to turn around stationary propensities is to focus on specific activities you can do each day.

2) Get a lot of exercises

Studies demonstrate that physical exercise expands the insulin affectability of cells when you exercise; less insulin is required to empower your blood glucose to enter your cells.

Numerous physical movement types decrease blood glucose levels in pre-diabetic grown-ups who are stout or overweight, counting vigorous exercise, quality preparing, and high-power stretch preparation.

One study of pre-diabetics showed that high-force exercise expanded insulin affectability by 85%... while tolerably extreme exercise expanded it by over half.

However, this impact just occurred when they worked out.

Another study found that to improve insulin reaction in pre-diabetics, they expected to consume in any event 2,000 calories per week through exercise. That isn't too difficult to think about doing if you set your focus on it.

Try to locate a physical action you appreciate and can usually embrace, and afterward stick to it as long as possible.

3) Quit Smoking

Other than tumors of the lung, breast, prostate, colon, throat, and stomach related tract, just as emphysema and coronary illness, research shows that there are proven connections between smoking (and introduction to recycled smoke) and type 2 diabetes.

Smoking builds the danger of diabetes by 44% in regular smokers and 61% in overwhelming smokers (more than 20 cigarettes every day), contrasted with non-smokers as per a meta-investigation of a few studies that together secured more than one million smokers.

Stopping smoking diminishes this hazard after some time, but not right away.

An investigation of moderately aged male smokers shows that five years in the wake of stopping their danger of developing diabetes was decreased by 13%. After 20 years, it was equivalent to individuals who had never smoked.

4) Lose Weight

Most individuals who develop type 2 diabetes are overweight or hefty. Also, individuals with pre-diabetes will, in general, have visceral fat, i.e., they haul their excess weight around their center and stomach organs, for example, the liver.

Studies have demonstrated that increased visceral fat advances insulin opposition, expanding the danger of diabetes significantly. This hazard can be diminished by shedding pounds, particularly around the center.

One investigation of more than 1,000 individuals found that for each kilogram (2.2 lbs.) they lost; their danger of diabetes was decreased by 16%. This examination additionally found that the most extreme decrease of a hazard was 96%, i.e., lost 6 kilograms

(13.2 lbs.).

There are numerous sound ways of shedding pounds by exercise and dieting.

You have numerous dietary alternatives to browse Mediterranean, paleo, low-carb, vegan. The best, maybe, is the Beating-Diabetes diet.

5)   Reduce the Fat in your Diet

As you know, the primary driver of type 2 diabetes is fat gumming up the receptors in your muscle cells, so the insulin can't open the cell films to permit glucose to enter. The "fix" is to unblock the receptors.

As you are pre-diabetic, fat is now starting to gum up the receptors. You can unblock the receptors by limiting the fat you ingest in your diet.

To limit the fat you eat:

- Make sure that under 10% of the content in any food you eat originates from fat (read the marks), and

- Reduce your utilization of meat, eggs, and dairy items, as reasonable, and center around foods dependent on plants (products of the soil).

- *It's that simple.*

 8

6) Reduce the Refined Carbs you eat

Refined starches are refined sugar and grain items that have been processed. The procedure removes dietary fiber, nutrients, and minerals from the grains.

Instances of refined carbs incorporate white sugar, granulated sugar, high fructose corn syrup, etc., just as white flour, white rice, white pasta, and so on. These are processed more quickly than complex starches.

Numerous investigations have indicated a connection between the constant utilization of sugar or other refined carbs and the danger of diabetes.

For instance, an examination that checked an aggregate of 37 investigations found that people with the most consumption of refined carbs are 40% more likely to develop diabetes than those with the least consumption.

This is because straightforward sugars and refined carbs are processed rapidly and are consumed quickly in the circulation system—this results in a spike in the degree of glucose in your blood.

However, as you are pre-diabetic, your body's cells are impervious to the activity of insulin. Therefore, the glucose spike invigorates your pancreas to deliver more insulin.

After some time, this prompts more elevated blood glucose and insulin levels in your blood until you develop out and out diabetes.

To keep away from this, you must stop placing sugar in your tea and espresso and quit drinking soft drinks and other sweet beverages.

You additionally need to begin eating regular foods, for example, entire grains, vegetables, organic products, and uncooked vegetables, which are all top hotspots for complex starches.

7) Eat a High Fiber Diet

Dietary fiber is the unpalatable bit of plant foodstuffs. There are two types of fiber and eating a lot of the two types is pivotal for forestalling pre-diabetes.

Solvent fiber will be a fiber that disintegrates in water to form a gooey gel-like material that eases back the rate at which food is ingested, lessening the probability of unexpected spikes in blood glucose.

Insoluble fiber can't disintegrate in water; however, it assimilates water, which makes your stool increasingly firm, facilitating its passing. It also is connected to decreases in blood glucose; however, how it functions isn't clear.

The primary sources of solvent fiber are vegetables (beans, peas, etc.) grains (oats, rye, and barley) vegetables, for example, broccoli, carrot and artichokes root vegetables, for example, yams and onions... also, the fleshy part of certain natural products, for example, prunes, plums, berries, bananas, apples, and pears.

10

Insoluble fiber is, for the most part, found in entire grains wheat and corn grain, nuts, seeds, potato skins, flax seeds. Also found in organic product, for example, avocados and bananas a few skins, for example, on tomatoes also, vegetables, for example, green beans, cauliflower, courgettes (zucchini) and celery.

A few plants contain significant measures of both dissolvable and insoluble fiber. Eating a lot of vegetables and foods grown from the ground will give you enough fiber to forestall your pre-diabetes developing into diabetes.

8) Minimize Your Consumption of Prepared foods

Prepared foods, for example, bacon, sausage, pâté, salami, breakfast oats, cheddar, tinned vegetables, bread, delicious tidbits (crisps, hotdog moves, pies, and pastries), cakes and rolls, microwave suppers, etc., are brimming with oils, including fats, included sugar, refined grains and a wide range of added substances.

Prepared foods are connected to a wide range of medical issues, including diabetes. One investigation found that low-quality diets that are high in processed foods increase the danger of diabetes by 30%.

So, to delay your diabetes developing into interminable diabetes, you have to decrease prepared foods. Eat vegetables, natural products, nuts, and other plant-based foods.

9) Restrict Partition Sizes

When food hits your stomach, everything begins to be processed on the double.

Along these lines, eating a lot at one sitting has been shown to cause higher glucose and insulin levels in pre-diabetic individuals.

A two-year investigation of pre-diabetic men found that the individuals who reduced the quantity of food they ate in one supper had a 46% lower danger of developing diabetes contrasted with the individuals who kept on eating huge amounts.

Another investigation of individuals with pre-diabetes inferred that the individuals who practiced portion control brought down their blood glucose and insulin levels significantly in the following 12 weeks.

Along these lines, to forestall the beginning of diabetes, you have to practice portion control.

10) Drink Lots of Water, Coffee and Tea

Drinking lots of water should be your essential drink.

Sticking with water more often means that you will keep away from drinks that are high in sugar, additives, and other harmful ingredients.

A massive observational investigation of 2,800 individuals found that the individuals who consumed multiple servings of sugar-improved drinks a day had a 99% increased danger of developing

LADA and a 20% higher risk of developing type 2 diabetes.

LADA, inactive immune system diabetes of grown-ups, is a type of type 1 diabetes that happens in individuals more than 18 years old.

A few studies have discovered that expanded water utilization (as opposed to increasing the number of soft drinks or natural product juices you devour) prompts better blood glucose control and insulin reaction.

One 24-week study, for instance, demonstrated that overweight grown-ups who changed diet soft drinks for water as a significant aspect of a health improvement plan encountered a reduction in insulin opposition and lower levels of blood glucose and insulin in the wake of fasting.

So, drink a lot of water, at any rate, 2 to 4 liters, a day to stop diabetes developing.

Ensure you stay away from the sugar-filled soft drinks and caffeinated drinks. Instead, when you need a boost, go for coffee or tea.

Coffee and tea contain polyphenols, cancer prevention agents that may secure against diabetes. Green tea additionally contains epigallocatechin gallate (EGCG), one of a kind of cancer prevention agents that has been shown to decrease the production of glucose from the liver and to build insulin affectability.

A few investigations have indicated that drinking coffee

consistently decreases the danger of type 2 diabetes by somewhere in the range of 8 to 54%. The best decrease in chance is found in the individuals who drink the most.

An examination of a few investigations, which included tea just as much as coffee, discovered comparative outcomes. This survey additionally demonstrated that the danger of developing diabetes was decreased the most in ladies (everything being equal) and overweight men.

So, it's a lot of water, tea, and coffee for pre-diabetics who wish to abstain from developing diabetes.

11) Take Day by Day Healthy Enhancements

Nutrition enhancement covers smaller scale supplements, for example, nutrients, dietary minerals, and unsaturated fats.

Vitamins are crucial for wellbeing. All nutrients can be categorized as one of two primary types, water-solvent or fat-dissolvable.

Water-dissolvable nutrients are on the whole of the B vitamins, besides vitamin C. These nutrients are not put away in your body, and you dispose of abundant amounts in your urine. Consequently, they can't develop toxic levels in your body.

Fat-solvent are vitamins A, D, E, and K. To ingest these vitamins, you need an amount of fat in your diet. Any excess amounts are put away in your body tissues so they could, hypothetically, develop to dangerous levels. In any case, this is incredibly uncommon.

Minerals are partitioned into two types, significant minerals and trace minerals.

Significant minerals are the minerals you need in measures of 100 milligrams (mg) or more every day. These minerals are calcium, phosphorus, magnesium, sulfur, potassium, sodium, and chloride.

Trace minerals are required in measures of fewer than 100mg every day. Trace minerals incorporate iron, iodine, zinc, fluoride, selenium, copper, chromium, manganese, and molybdenum.

Minerals are used in an assortment of functions. For instance, your body uses calcium to make bones and teeth, and iron to make the hemoglobin in your red platelets.

Although, everything being equal and dietary minerals are not yet entirely understood by researchers, and even though the results of clinical tests regularly contradict one another, day by day dietary enhancement should help forestall your pre-diabetes developing into diabetes.

This is what you must take every day:

- Multivitamin: to ensure all your dietary needs are secured.

- Vitamin B12 (4mcg) in a different tablet: for the wellbeing of your sensory system as your pre-diabetes is probably going to be influencing your nerves as of now.

- Calcium (400mg) in addition to vitamin D (2.5mcg) together in a different tablet to guarantee the soundness of your bones.

- High-quality cod-liver oil capsule with vitamins D and E, in a different capsule: to ensure you ingest sufficient measures of the essential unsaturated fats omega three and omega 6.

There is an accentuation on vitamin D because this vitamin is significant for adequate power over your blood glucose.

An assortment of studies shows that people who have too little vitamin D in their circulation system are at more danger of all types of diabetes. One examination found that people with the most significant levels of vitamin D in their blood were 43% less likely to develop diabetes contrasted with people with the least levels.

Most wellbeing associations suggest keeping up a vitamin D blood level of at any rate 75nmol/l (30ng/ml).

Controlled investigations have demonstrated that when individuals who lack vitamin D take supplements, their blood glucose levels are standardized, and their danger of developing diabetes is diminished significantly.

12) Add Characteristic Herbs to Your Diet

The web is loaded with claims, for the most part, fake, that specific herbs can prevent your pre-diabetes from developing into the all-out form of the disease. Here are a couple of the more believable cases:

- **Cinnamon**: is a profoundly sweet-smelling zest with an exceptionally particular flavor. It is used in conventional medicine to treat an assortment of ailments, obviously with some success.

Reports on the web recommend that cinnamon can cut fasting glucose levels by up to 30%, so I started sprinkling one enormous teaspoon on my porridge (oats) in the first part of the day. Inside a couple of days, my normal glucose levels on getting up had dropped by almost 0.5mmol/l (9mg/l) or about 8%, a considerable amount shy of 30% a significant decrease in any case.

So, I can't help suspecting that this zest, as ground powder you can purchase from your nearby general store, can help you improve your blood glucose levels and, accordingly, help prevent your pre-diabetes developing into diabetes. Bitter melon... otherwise known as harsh gourd or karela (in India), is a one of a kind vegetable-natural product that can be used as a food or medicine. It is frequently suggested for the control of diabetes.

Various clinical examinations have indicated that bitter melon is successful in improving blood glucose levels, expanding the discharge of insulin, and diminishing insulin obstruction.

In January 2011, for instance, the results of a four-week clinical trial were published in the Journal of Ethnopharmacology, which indicated that a 2,000 mg everyday portion of bitter melon significantly decreased blood glucose levels among patients with type 2 diabetes. Anyway, the hypoglycemic impact was not as much as that of a 1,000 mg for an every day portion of metformin, a well-known diabetes drug.

Even though it might be of some assistance in preventing your pre-diabetes deteriorating, the bitter melon should be treated with care as it has been related to unnatural birth cycles and actuated premature births in animals. Therefore, it ought to be kept away from if you are pregnant or need to get pregnant.

- **Curcumin**: is a part of turmeric, one of the fundamental ingredients in curries. It has anti-inflammatory properties and has been used in Ayurvedic medicine for quite a long time.

Research shows that curcumin can help decrease significant markers in people with pre-diabetes.

In a controlled 9-month investigation of 240 pre-diabetic grown-ups, none of the individuals who took 750mg of curcumin every day developed diabetes, yet over 16% of the benchmark group did. The investigation additionally noticed that insulin affectability among the individuals who took curcumin expanded, as did the working of their insulin-creating cells in the pancreas.

In this way, the advantages of curcumin in diminishing insulin opposition and lessening the hazard that pre-diabetics will develop out and out diabetes have all the earmarks of being very much demonstrated.

- **Berberine**: is an alkaloid extricated from different plants used in customary Chinese medicine. It is demonstrated to be mitigating and effective against diabetic impacts. It works by lessening the creation of glucose in the liver and expanding insulin affectability.

An amalgamation of 14 investigations of human and animal research has demonstrated that 1,500mg of berberine, taken in three dosages of 500mg each, is similarly effective as taking 1,500mg of metformin or 4mg glibenclamide, two well-known pharmaceuticals for treating type 2 diabetes. Berberine is one of only a handful of many supplements demonstrated to be as powerful as ordinary diabetes drugs.

Berberine, in any case, can react with different drugs and caution should be exercised... ask your primary care physician before you attempt to use it to forestall your pre-diabetes deteriorating.

- *Admonition (1):* Spurious cases that specific supplements can fix or forestall sicknesses flourish on the web. Anyway, there are a couple of reliable sources that contain research-tried data. These are for the most part associated with respectable colleges, clinical schools and teaching medical clinics.

- **Admonition (2):** Some herbs and supplements may combine with your diabetes prescription (counting insulin) and cause too low blood glucose. So, check with your primary care physician before using them.

BREAKFAST RECIPES

MINI VEGGIE QUICHE

A Veggie Diabetic Friendly Recipe. These are mini quiches that can also be called 'Stand Alone Meal'. It's easy to always have a delicious breakfast - ready to go. They are a great weekend recipe you can prepare for the family. You would love this meal because they freeze so well, and they can be served with a light salad and any of your favorite drink.

Enjoy!

INGREDIENTS

- 9 eggs
- 8 ounces of chopped spinach
- 1 small red pepper, chopped
- 1 cup of milk
- 1 cup of shredded cheddar
- 1/2 teaspoon of salt
- 1 small red onion, chopped
- Butter

PREPARATIONS

- In a large sauté pan, add a tablespoon of butter and melt it over a medium low heat.
- Add in the onions and cook until just translucent, for about 2 minutes.
- Add in the spinach and cook until it's wilted.
- Add the red peppers and more butter if needed.

21

- Sauté for about 1 minute and set it aside.

- Grease a muffin pan that holds 12 muffins.

- Divide the sautéed veggies between the tins.

- In a large mixing bowl, crack the 9 eggs and add in the milk and salt. Whisk together.

- Divide half of the cheddar cheese between the muffin tins.

- Then divide the egg mixture.

- Bake for about 10 minutes at 375 degrees F.

- Remove from heat and divide the rest of the cheddar, topping the quiches.

- Place it back into the oven and bake until the eggs are set. You can use toothpick to check.

- Remove from heat and let it cool.

- Serve and enjoy.

NOTE:

The mini quiches keep well in an air-tight container in the fridge for 3 to 4 days. You can easily reheat them in the oven (at 350 °F/180 °C for about 10 to 15 minutes) or in the microwave (on the high setting for 1 to 2 minutes).

PREP TIME: 15 mins

COOK TIME: 15 mins

TOTAL TIME: 30 mins

YIELD: 12 mini quiches

SHAKSHUKA

This kind of recipe is loaded with spices, eggs and tomato sauce. It's so easy to prepare and can be ready-to-eat within 30 to 40 minutes.

Using canned tomatoes for this shakshuka will be so easy (though you can always use your fresh tomatoes - it's not a problem). You don't have to worry too much because it's a healthy and diabetic friendly recipe you can always have in a bright morning.

INGREDIENTS

- 4 garlic cloves, finely chopped
- 2 teaspoons of paprika
- 1 teaspoon of cumin
- 1 medium onion, diced
- 1 red bell pepper, deseeded and diced
- 1/4 teaspoon of chili powder
- 1 28-ounces can of whole peeled tomatoes
- 1 small bunch of fresh cilantro, chopped
- 1 small bunch of fresh parsley, chopped
- 6 large eggs
- salt and pepper, to taste

PREPARATIONS

- In a large sauté pan, heat olive oil on medium heat.

- Add the chopped onion and bell pepper. Then cook until the onion becomes translucent, for about 5 minutes.

- Add spices and garlic, then cook for another minute.

- Pour the juice and can of tomatoes into the pan, then use a large spoon to break down the tomatoes.

- Season with pepper and salt and bring the sauce to a simmer.

- Make small wells in the sauce using a large spoon and crack the eggs into each well.

- Cover the pan and cook until the eggs are done to your liking, for about 5 to 8 minutes.

- Garnish with parsley and chopped cilantro.

- Serve and enjoy.

NOTE:

Shakshuka can be stored in the fridge for up to 1 week or can be frozen. To serve, warm in a pan with a little oil and top with the cheese / nuts / herbs.

PREP TIME: 10 mins

COOK TIME: 20 mins

TOTAL TIME: 30 mins

YIELD: 6 servings

HEALTHY GRANOLA

Healthy Granola is truly the best granola recipe! It's so easy and quick to make. It's delicious and flavorful and it's naturally sweetened with maple syrup. You can add in some possible variations to spice it up like dried fruit, chocolate chips and peanut butter or any other spices that you love.

Have this meal for your breakfast and be happy for the rest of the day!

INGREDIENTS

- 2 teaspoons of ground cinnamon
- 3/4 teaspoon of fine sea salt
- 1/2 cup of melted coconut oil
- 4 cups of old-fashioned oats
- 2/3 cup of unsweetened coconut flakes (or 1/2 cup of shredded coconut)
- 1 cup of slivered almonds (or your preferred kind of seeds/nuts)
- 1/4 cup of chia seeds (optional)
- 1/3 cup of maple syrup
- 2 teaspoons of vanilla extract
- 1/2 cup of chopped dried fruit or semisweet chocolate chips (optional)

PREPARATIONS

- Heat oven to 350 degrees F.

- Use parchment paper to line a large baking sheet and set it aside.

- Stir together almonds, oats, cinnamon and sea salt in a large mixing bowl until evenly combined.

- Stir together the maple syrup, melted coconut oil and vanilla extract in a separate measuring cup until well combined.

- Pour the coconut oil mixture into the oats mixture.

- Stir until evenly combined.

- Spread the granola out on the prepared baking sheet.

- Bake, stirring once halfway through, for about 20 minutes.

- Remove from the oven and add the coconut and stir the mixture well.

- Bake until the granola is lightly golden and toasted, for about 5 more minutes.

- Remove from the oven, then transfer to a wire baking rack.

- Let it cool till the granola reaches room temp.

- Then stir in the chocolate chips, dried fruit or any other optional add-ins you might prefer.

- Serve immediately or store in an airtight container at room temp.

- Enjoy.

NOTE:

You can absolutely preserve granola bars. You wrap the bars individually first with waxed paper or parchment paper, then store in large, labeled Ziploc bags. They freeze well for up to 2 months. To thaw, just pull out how many granola bars you want out of the freezer and leave them on the counter for 30 minutes.

PREP TIME: 10 mins

COOK TIME: 25 mins

TOTAL TIME: 35 mins

YIELD: 6 cups

CINNAMON OATMEAL MUFFINS WITH APPLE

Cinnamon Oatmeal Muffins are make-ahead comforting healthy recipe for people with Diabetics. They are awesome and can be packaged as snacks as well.

You can swap the apples for strawberries or blueberries and they have a subtle sweetness that makes a nutritious and delicious breakfast option for kids and adults as well. You need to try these muffins.

INGREDIENTS

Topping:

- 1 tablespoon of melted butter
- 1/4 cup of quick-cooking oats
- 1 tablespoon of brown sugar
- 1/4 teaspoon of ground cinnamon

Muffins:

- 1 - 1/2 teaspoons of ground cinnamon
- 1 teaspoon of baking powder
- 1 egg, lightly beaten
- 1 teaspoon of vanilla extract
- 1/2 teaspoon of baking soda
- 1/2 teaspoon of salt
- 1 1/2 cups of quick-cooking oats

- 1 1/4 cups of all-purpose flour
- 2 tablespoons of all-purpose flour
- 1/2 cup of brown sugar
- 1/2 cup of unsweetened applesauce
- 1/2 cup of milk
- 1/4 cup of vegetable oil
- 1 apple chopped, peeled and cored

PREPARATIONS

- Preheat oven to 400 degrees F.
- Grease a 12-cup muffin tin and line with paper liners.
- Stir 1 tablespoon of brown sugar, 1/4 cup of oats, 1/4 teaspoon of cinnamon and melted butter together in a small bowl. Set it aside.
- Whisk 1/2 cup of brown sugar, 1 1/2 cups of oats, flour, baking powder, 1 1/2 teaspoons of cinnamon, salt and baking soda together in a large bowl.
- Stir milk, applesauce, oil, egg and vanilla extract together in a bowl.
- Stir applesauce mixture into flour mixture just until all ingredients are moistened.
- Stir in the apple and spoon of apple mixture into prepared muffins cups, for about 2/3 full, sprinkle oat and top mixture evenly over each muffin.
- Bake in the preheated oven, for about 15 minutes until a toothpick inserted near the center comes out clean.
- Serve and enjoy.

NOTE:

Bake the oatmeal cups, cool completely, and store in the refrigerator all week for easy breakfasts. Reheat in the microwave or bake in a 350°F (177°C) oven for 5 - 6 minutes. To freeze, bake and cool oatmeal cups. Cover tightly and freeze for up to 3 months. Thaw in the refrigerator or at room temperature. Warm to your liking.

PREP TIME: 20 mins

COOK TIME: 15 mins

TOTAL TIME: 35 mins

YIELD: 12 muffins

VEGGIE OMELET

Veggie Omelet is one of the easiest and fastest breakfast recipes to eat. It is essential to start your day off right with nutrient-dense vegetables and protein.

This recipe can be prepared and eaten as a side dish or as a full meal. It's so healthy, simply delicious, light and fluffy.

The most interesting part of it is that you can use your favorite vegetables to create your own perfect omelet.

INGREDIENTS

- 4 eggs
- 2 tablespoons of milk
- 3/4 teaspoon of salt
- 2 tablespoons of butter
- 1 small onion, chopped
- 1 green bell pepper, chopped
- 1/8 teaspoon of freshly ground black pepper
- 2 ounces of shredded Swiss cheese

PREPARATIONS

- In a medium skillet, melt 1 tablespoon of butter over medium heat.
- Place bell pepper and onion inside the skillet.
- Cook until vegetables are just tender, for about 5 minutes, stirring occasionally.

- Beat the eggs with 1/2 teaspoon of salt and pepper with milk while the vegetables are cooking.

- In a small bowl, shred the cheese and set it aside.

- Remove the vegetables from the heat.

- Transfer them into a separate bowl and sprinkle the rest of the salt over them.

- Melt the rest of the butter over medium heat.

- Coat the skillet with the butter.

- Add the egg mixture while the butter is bubbly and cook the egg until the eggs begin to set on the bottom of the pan, for about 2 minutes.

- Lift the edges of the omelet gently using a spatula to let the uncooked part of the eggs flows to the edges and cook.

- Continue cooking until the center of the omelet starts to look dry, for about 3 minutes.

- Sprinkle the cheese over the omelet.

- Spoon the vegetable mixture into the center of the omelet.

- Using a spatula gently fold one edge of the omelet, over the vegetables,

- Let the omelet cook until the cheese melts to your desired consistency, for about 2 minutes.

- Slide the omelet out of the skillet and place on a plate.

- Cut into half, serve and enjoy.

NOTE:

Freezer bags are a great option for preserving omelets in either the fridge of the freezer. Store omelets in the fridge for only about 3-4 days. Omelets should be tightly wrapped or sealed in an airtight container or bag. The key to storing them is to make sure they are sealed tightly into whatever storage format you use.

You can preserve omelets by storing it in the freezer for up to 4 months. They will taste the freshest if they are used within 2 months. To store in the freezer, wrap tightly or place into freezer bags or an airtight container. This is just to ensure that they really are sealed tight in the order to preserve the flavor.

PREP TIME: 10 mins

COOK TIME: 15 mins

TOTAL TIME: 25 mins

YIELD: 2 servings

EGG PEPPER CUPS

All you will be needing are eggs, fresh ground pepper, whatever fresh herbs you have on hand and some coloured bell peppers to get your morning meal ready. This is the kind of recipe that is so simple to make-ahead and can be ready to eat within 30 minutes.

Giving this Eggs Pepper Cups a try would be great seriously. An easy breakfast idea that is full of filling protein to take on your day. I call it a morning

energizer.

INGREDIENTS

- 4 large eggs
- Freshly ground pepper and kosher salt
- 4 small multicolored bell peppers
- Chopped fresh herbs

PREPARATIONS

- Preheat oven to 350 degrees F.
- Slice bottom of 2-inches of the pepper (do this for each of the pepper - in 1 piece) to form shallow cups.
- Reserve tops for another use next time.
- Place the pepper on a baking sheet.
- Crack 1 egg into each of the pepper.
- Season with pepper and salt.

- Bake for about 25 minutes, until yolks are still a little runny and whites are firm.

- Sprinkle with chopped fresh herbs of your choice.

- Serve and enjoy.

NOTES:

Keep them all in an airtight container in the refrigerator or place each individual egg muffin cup in a resealable bag for an easy grab-and-go breakfast. Dispose after 6 days. You can also freeze the cooked egg muffins, once cooled, in a resealable bag for up to 3 months.

PREP TIME: 5 mins

COOK TIME: 0 mins

TOTAL TIME: 30 mins

YIELD: 6 pepper cups

VEGGIE FRITTATA

MY **BONUS** RECIPE

Veggie Frittata is just like an open omelet that sure makes a colorful presentation. They are vegetarian meals that are a great way to transform eggs into a more substantial breakfast. You should know that Eggs are naturally rich in protein and low in carbs. So, I believe this is the perfect combo to maintain steady blood-sugar levels.

Start your day with this delicious meal today and enjoy.

INGREDIENTS

- 6 eggs
- 1/4 cup of cilantro chopped
- 1/2 cup of cherry tomatoes sliced
- 1/4 cup of full fat yogurt optional
- 1 cup of mushrooms chopped
- 8-10 stalks asparagus ends trimmed and chopped
- 1 cup of shredded mozzarella cheese divided
- 1/4 cup of red onions chopped

PREPARATIONS

- Preheat the oven to 425 degrees F.
- Whisk together the egg, salt, pepper, half of the shredded mozzarella cheese and yogurt; set mixture aside.
- In a cast iron pan or oven safe pan, heat the olive oil.

- Add mushrooms, onions and asparagus and cook until the vegetables soften for about 5 minutes.

- Pour the egg mixture on top of the cooked vegetables.

- Place sliced cherry tomatoes on top, then add the rest of the cheese.

- Bake in the preheated oven uncovered for about 15 minutes until the center is set and not jiggly.

- Serve and enjoy.

NOTE:

Frittata can be preserved well for a few days in the refrigerator. You can serve leftover frittata chilled, let it come to room temperature on its own, or gently warm individual slices in the microwave or oven.

PREP TIME: 10 mins

COOK TIME: 15 mins

TOTAL TIME: 25 mins

YIELD: 4 servings

COCONUT PORRIDGE

MY **BONUS** RECIPE

According to the medical website WebMD, coconut porridge could help to control blood sugar in diabetes patients. It's better at maintaining blood sugar levels over a longer period of time. It's a food that takes longer to digest and the kind of foods that takes longer to digest are extremely better for diabetes.

Coconut Porridge is one of the most nutritious breakfast dishes you can serve for your entire family in the morning. *Enjoy your morning.*

INGREDIENTS

- 1 ounce of coconut oil or butter
- 4 tablespoons of coconut cream
- 1 beaten egg
- 1 pinch of salt
- 1 tablespoon of coconut flour
- 1 pinch of ground psyllium husk powder

PREPARATIONS

- Combine the coconut flour, egg, psyllium husk powder and salt in a small bowl.
- Melt the butter and coconut cream over low heat.

- Whisk in the egg mixture slowly, combining until you achieve a thick creamy texture.

- Serve with cream or coconut milk.

- Top your porridge with some fresh or frozen berries.

- Serve and enjoy.

NOTE:

Store into lidded containers in the refrigerator for up to 3 days.

PREP TIME: 10 mins

COOK TIME: 0 mins

TOTAL TIME: 10 mins

YIELD: 1 serving

LUNCH RECIPES

TORTILLA CHICKEN SOUP

This recipe delivers the same flavor you love in traditional tortilla soup, but without all high carbs ingredients.

It's so good and perfect for people with diabetics. You can top with crispy tortilla chips and lighten this up by baking the tortilla so you can have heartier recipe. I would suggest you should add lime to give it a zesty freshness. Also, this recipe is for you if you're looking forwards to eating healthy.

INGREDIENTS

- 1 cup of corn, drained if canned
- 2 chicken breasts boneless, skinless
- 1/4 cup of cilantro chopped
- 1 lime juiced
- 1 sliced avocado
- 1 tablespoon of olive oil
- 1 chopped onion
- 3 large cloves garlic, minced
- 1 jalapeño deseeded and diced
- 1 teaspoon of ground cumin
- 1 teaspoon of chili powder
- 14.5 ounces of crushed tomatoes
- 1 can diced tomatoes with chilies

- 3 cups of chicken broth
- 14.5 ounce can black beans, drained and rinsed

Crispy Tortilla Strips

- 1/4 cup of olive oil
- salt
- 6 6-inches corn tortillas cut into 1/4-inch strips

PREPARATIONS

- Over medium high heat, heat 1/4 cup of olive oil in a small pan.
- Add tortilla strips into small batches and then fry till crisp.
- Drain and add sprinkle salt.
- In a large pot over medium heat, heat olive oil and add garlic, onion, jalapeno and onion, then cook until softened.
- Add the rest of the ingredients and simmer until chicken is cooked through, for about 20 minutes.
- Remove chicken and shred it.
- Add it back to the pot and then simmer for just 3 mins.
- Spoon your soup into bowls.
- Top with lime wedges, tortilla strips and sliced avocado.
- Serve and enjoy.

NOTE:

This chicken tortilla soup recipe is perfect for freezing, because it doesn't contain dairy and reheats really well. Cool the soup down completely, then store in a freezer-safe container. It will last in the refrigerator for 3-4 days in an airtight container. To reheat, pour into a saucepan over medium-low heat, stirring until warmed through.

PREP TIME: 10 mins

COOK TIME: 30 mins

TOTAL TIME: 40 mins

YIELD: 8 servings

CHICKEN BROCCOLI SALAD

Chicken Broccoli Salad is just so easy, creamy and simple to make. This healthy meal is the best for you if you're a veggie fan. It is super nutritious and amazingly versatile too. You should ideally keep a safe distance from junk and processed foods if you are a diabetes patient. It is also advisable to avoid sugary foods. This is why I'm introducing this Chicken Broccoli Salad to you.

Enjoy!

INGREDIENTS

- 1/4 cup of apple cider vinegar
- 1/4 cup of white sugar
- 1/4 cup of crumbled cooked bacon
- 8 cups of broccoli florets
- 3 cooked skinless, boneless chicken breast halves, cubed
- 1 cup of chopped walnuts
- 6 green onions, chopped
- 1 cup of mayonnaise

PREPARATIONS

- Combine chicken, broccoli, walnuts and green onions in a large bowl.
- Whisk together vinegar, mayonnaise and sugar in a bowl until it's well blended.

- Pour mayonnaise dressing over broccoli mixture and toss to coat.

- Cover and refrigerate till chilled if you feel like.

- To serve: sprinkle with crumbled bacon.

- Serve and enjoy.

NOTE:

Store, covered, in refrigerator until ready to serve, so that the dressing has time to chill and the flavors blend. The broccoli salad can be kept, covered, in the refrigerator for several days.

PREP TIME: 15 mins

COOK TIME: 0 mins

TOTAL TIME: 1 hour 15 mins

YIELD: 10 servings

BLACK BEAN SALAD

You need to have a taste of different salad every day. This Black Bean Salad is a very tasty and satisfying lunch salad. I love this combination of veggies and beans. It's a complete meal that is tasty, healthy and super easy to make.

The most interesting part of this meal is its excellent when cold or heated. *So good!*

INGREDIENTS

- 1 avocado, deseeded, peeled and cut into chunks
- 1/2 to 1 teaspoon of sugar (to taste)
- Salt and pepper to taste
- 1/2 cup of chopped fresh cilantro
- 1 1/2 cups of freshly cooked black beans (or 1 (15 ounces) can of black beans, drained and rinsed)
- 1 1/2 cups of frozen corn, defrosted (or fresh corn, drained, parboiled and cooled, or cooled and grilled)
- 1/2 cup of shallots or chopped green onions (including onion greens)
- 2 tablespoons of lime juice (about the juice from one lime)
- 1 tablespoon of extra virgin olive oil
- 1/2 fresh jalapeño pepper, minced and deseeded, or 1/2 pickled jalapeño pepper, minced (not seeded)
- 3 fresh plum tomatoes, deseeded and chopped and/or 1 red bell pepper, chopped and deseeded

PREPARATIONS

- Combine the corn, black beans, minced jalapenos, chopped green onions, chopped tomatoes or red bell pepper, olive oil and lime juice in a large bowl.

- Fold in the chopped avocado gently.

- Add pepper and salt to taste.

- Sprinkle with sugar to taste (sugar that is enough to balance the acidity from the lime juice).

- Chill before serving.

- Add the chopped fresh cilantro.

- Serve and enjoy.

NOTE:

To preserve, refrigerate the bean salad in airtight containers. Properly stored, bean salad will last for 3 to 5 days in the refrigerator.

PREP TIME: 20 mins

COOK TIME: 0 mins

TOTAL TIME: 20 mins

YIELD: 6 servings

KALE SALAD WITH LEMON DRESSING

This is a vegetarian, low-carb salad that might not sound like a filling meal, but this is loaded with leafy greens and protein that will power you through your day. As we all know, kale is one of those foods that is incredibly healthy, but most people are always afraid to try. Taking a step to try this recipe is a great way to get more vegetables into your diet. This Kale Salad with Lemon Dressing is delicious and actually easy to prepare.

INGREDIENTS

Lemon Dressing

- 1 minced garlic clove
- 1 teaspoon of dried oregano
- 1/2 cup of extra virgin olive oil
- 1/4 cup of lemon juice
- Salt and pepper to taste

Kale Salad

- 1/2 red onion thinly sliced
- 1/2 cup of crumbled feta cheese
- 1-pint cherry or grape tomatoes halved
- 1 large bunch of about 10 ounces (or 3-4 cups of kale leaves), finely chopped
- 1 cucumber deseeded and diced

PREPARATIONS

Making the Lemon Dressing:

- Combine together the lemon juice, garlic, olive oil, salt, oregano and pepper in a small or medium mixing bowl.

- Whisk until well combined.

Making the Kale Salad:

- Add together all the chopped ingredients in a large bowl and combine.

- Pour the dressing over the salad and mix together.

- Sprinkle with some feta cheese just before serving.

- You can store your dressed and prepared salad in the fridge for up to 2 days.

- Serve and enjoy.

NOTE:

You can store this salad in an airtight container in the fridge for up to 7 days.

PREP TIME: 10 mins

COOK TIME: 0 mins

TOTAL TIME: 10 mins

YIELD: 4 servings

CARROT GINGER SOUP

Carrot Ginger Soup is an easy make-ahead meal and a great way to add some fiber-packed and nutritious vegetables to your diet. If you have diabetes, the more vegetables you eat, the better. This meal is low in carbs and calories, which is a must have for people with diabetes.

It's full of lots of the good stuff your body needs, such as vitamins, antioxidants, minerals and even fiber. This meal does not only offer fragrance and color but it's light and soothing as well.

INGREDIENTS

- 1 tablespoon of apple cider vinegar
- 3 to 4 cups of vegetable broth
- Sea salt and fresh black pepper
- 1 tablespoon of extra-virgin olive oil
- 1 cup of chopped yellow onions
- 3 garlic cloves, smashed
- 2 heaping cups of chopped carrots
- 1 - 1/2 teaspoons of grated fresh ginger
- 1 teaspoon of maple syrup, or to taste (optional)
- coconut milk for garnish, optional
- dollops of pesto, optional

PREPARATIONS

- In a large pot, heat the olive oil over medium heat.

- Add the onions and a pinch of salt and pepper.

- Cook until softened, stirring occasionally, for about 8 minutes.

- Add the smashed garlic cloves and the chopped carrots into the pot.

- Cook for another 8 minutes, stirring occasionally.

- Stir in the ginger and add the apple cider vinegar.

- The next thing you'll want to do is add 3 to 4 cups of broth.

- Reduce to a simmer and cook for about 30 minutes, until the carrots are soft.

- Let it cool slightly and transfer into a blender.

- Blend until smooth.

- Taste and adjust seasonings.

- Add maple syrup if you feel like.

- Serve with a dollop of pesto or drizzle of coconut milk.

- Enjoy.

NOTE:

Leftover carrot ginger soup can be frozen for a quick and simple meal later. Although creamed soups sometimes separate when you defrost and reheat them due to the cream base, it can be remedied with careful blending. If you're freezing the soup, let it cool to room temperature and then transfer it too quart-sized freezer bags (the sturdy ones please). Freeze these flat and then they stack nicely in your fridge. Reheating the soup is easy. Let it thaw slowly or dunk it in warm water for a faster thaw.

PREP TIME: 15 mins

COOK TIME: 30 mins

TOTAL TIME: 45 mins

YIELD: 4 servings

SHRIMP SALAD

Shrimp salad is a perfect light lunch. Loaded with healthy ingredients like black pepper, onion, celery and kosher salt. I'm sure it combines all of your favorite ingredients in one bowl, right?

This is a satisfying dish that has all of the crunch with much less fat. When you have a bite, you bite into a perfectly crispy shrimp salad.

INGREDIENTS

For the Salad:

- Freshly ground black pepper
- 1/4 finely chopped red onion
- 1 finely chopped stalk celery
- 1 pound of shrimp, deveined and peeled
- 1 tablespoon of extra-virgin olive oil
- Kosher salt
- 2 tablespoons of freshly chopped dill
- Toasted bread or butterhead or romaine lettuce, for serving

For the Dressing:

- 1/2 cup of mayonnaise
- Juice and zest of 1 lemon
- 1 teaspoon of Dijon mustard

PREPARATIONS

- Preheat oven to 400 degrees F.

- Toss shrimp with oil on a large baking sheet.

- Season with pepper and salt.

- Bake for about 5 minutes, until shrimp are completely opaque.

- Whisk together mayonnaise, zest, lemon juice and Dijon in a large bowl.

- Season with pepper and salt.

- Add your cooked shrimp, celery, red onion and dill to bowl.

- Then toss until well combined.

- Serve over lettuce and enjoy.

NOTE:

This will last up to 3 days in the fridge when preserved properly in an airtight container.

PREP TIME: 5 mins

COOK TIME: 0 mins

TOTAL TIME: 20 mins

YIELD: 2 servings

CRISPY TOFU

MY **BONUS** RECIPE

This is one of the best crispy tofu recipes for lunch. It uses little oil and it's baked to perfection. It can be perfect for just snacking on!

It's really easy to make, so crispy and it's made with healthy ingredients. The sesame oil used in this recipe gives it a very nice flavor (by the way, you can use avocado / olive oil - it's your choice).

I hope you'll enjoy it.

INGREDIENTS

- 1/4 teaspoon of garlic powder
- 1/4 teaspoon of pure maple syrup
- 1/4 teaspoon of rice wine vinegar
- 1 tablespoon of toasted sesame oil, or your favorite oil
- 1 (14 ounces) container extra firm tofu, pressed and patted dry for at least 15 minutes
- 1 teaspoon of soy sauce or tamari
- 2 teaspoons of corn starch or arrowroot powder

PREPARATIONS

- Preheat oven to 400 degrees F.
- Whisk together tamari or soy sauce, sesame oil, maple syrup, garlic powder and vinegar in a medium sized bowl.
- Cut the press tofu into bite sized pieces.

- Place the pieces into the oil mixture.

- Stir the tofu using a spoon or spatula, making sure it's completely coated.

- Sprinkle 1 teaspoon of the arrowroot powder over it and mix well till all of the tofu is coated.

- Sprinkle the rest of the arrowroot powder and mix carefully just until you can't see the dry white powder anymore.

- Using parchment paper or nonstick to line a large baking sheet.

- Pour the tofu onto baking sheet and arrange it so that the pieces won't be touching each other.

- Bake tofu until crispy and golden, for about 25 minutes, stirring 2 to 3 times during the baking.

- Let the tofu sit for some minutes to crisp even more before enjoying.

- Serve and enjoy.

NOTE:

While crispy tofu is slightly seasoned, it does still benefit from a sauce. Best when fresh but can be stored in the refrigerator for up to 3 days. Reheat in a 375 degrees F (190 C) oven until very hot.

PREP TIME: 15 mins

COOK TIME: 30 mins

TOTAL TIME: 35 mins

YIELD: 4 servings

SPINACH SOUP WITH PESTO & CHICKEN

MY **BONUS** RECIPE

This soup is from Italy. It's a fragrant flavored soup that takes advantage of quick cooking ingredients. It features a simple homemade pesto which adds a fresh herb flavor to the meal.

You can substitute about 3 tablespoons of store-bought pesto if you can't wait to prepare this meal. Prepare, serve and enjoy!

INGREDIENTS

- 1 large clove garlic, minced
- 1/8 cup of lightly packed fresh basil leaves
- Freshly ground pepper to taste
- 5 cups of reduced-sodium chicken broth
- 1 1/2 teaspoons of dried marjoram
- 6 ounces of baby spinach, coarsely chopped
- 2 teaspoons with 1 tablespoon of extra-virgin olive oil, divided
- 1/2 cup of carrot or diced red bell pepper
- 1 large boneless, skinless chicken breast (about 8 ounces), cut into quarters
- 1 15-ounces can of cannellini beans or great northern beans, rinsed
- 1/4 cup of grated Parmesan cheese

- 3/4 cup of plain or herbed multigrain croutons for garnish (optional)

PREPARATIONS

- In a large saucepan, heat 2 tablespoons of oil over medium high heat.

- Add carrot or bell pepper with chicken together.

- Cook, turning the chicken and stirring occasionally, for about 3 minutes, until the chicken begins to brown.

- Add garlic and cook, stirring, for another 1 minute.

- Stir in marjoram and broth.

- Bring to a boil over high heat and reduce the heat.

- Simmer, stirring occasionally, for about 5 minutes until the chicken is cooked through.

- Transfer the chicken pieces to a clean cutting board to cool using a slotted spoon.

- Add beans and spinach into the pot, then bring to a boil.

- Cook for 5 mins to blend the flavors.

- In a food processor, combine the parmesan, 1 tablespoon of oil, basil.

- Process until a coarse paste forms, adding a little water and scrape down the sides.

- Cut the chicken into small size pieces.

- Stir the pesto and chicken into the pot.

- Season with pepper and heat until it's hot.

- Garnish with croutons, if you feel like.

- Serve and enjoy.

NOTE:

Store in a clean container wrapped with paper towels for 3 to 5 days. Place it in the refrigerator in the crisp drawer to save the greens for up to ten days. Paper towels absorb the moisture and keep it fresh.

PREP TIME: 10 mins

COOK TIME: 20 mins

TOTAL TIME: 30 mins

YIELD: 5 servings

DINNER RECIPES

FRENCH LENTILS

This is one of my favorite Diabetic Dinner Recipes because it helps stabilize your blood sugar levels. French Lentils are full of complex carbs that can help you with 25% of protein if you have diabetes.

French Lentils also improves the flow of blood, prevents heart disease and protects the artery walls.

INGREDIENTS

- 2 1/4 cups of French lentils
- 3 tablespoons of olive or vegetable oil
- 1 teaspoon of dried or fresh thyme
- 3 bay leaves
- 1 tablespoon of kosher salt
- 1 onion, peeled and finely chopped
- 2 cloves garlic, peeled and finely chopped
- 1 carrot, peeled and finely chopped

PREPARATIONS

- Place a large saucepan over a medium heat and add oil.
- Add chopped vegetables when hot and sauté for about 5 to 10 minutes, until softened.
- Add lentils, 6 cups of water, thyme, salt and bay leaves.
- Bring to a boil and reduce to a fast simmer.
- Simmer for 20 to 25 minutes until they are tender and have absorbed most of the water.

- Drain any excess water after lentils have cooked, if necessary.

- Serve immediately and enjoy.

NOTE:

Properly stored, cooked lentils will last for 3 to 5 days in the refrigerator. Cooked lentils should be discarded if left out for more than 2 hours at room temperature.

PREP TIME: 15 mins

COOK TIME: 25 mins

TOTAL TIME: 40 mins

YIELD: 4 servings

CHICKEN FAJITAS

This is a delicious Chicken Fajitas recipe that is super great for a weeknight meal. They are loaded with lots of light ingredients, flavor and are perfect if you're following diabetes diet.

They are easy and quick to make, and cleanup is pretty fast too.

INGREDIENTS

- 2 teaspoons of fajita seasoning
- 1 green bell pepper, cut into strips
- 1 red bell pepper, cut into strips
- 1 clove garlic, minced
- 1 cup of sliced onion
- 2 boneless, skinless chicken breasts, cut into strips
- 4 low-carb whole wheat tortillas, warmed

PREPARATIONS

- Cooking spray to coat a large skillet.
- Cook garlic, bell peppers and onion over medium heat until tender, for about 6 to 8 minutes, stirring occasionally.
- Remove to a plate.
- Add chicken and fajita seasoning; cook until no longer pink in center, for about 5 minutes.
- Return vegetables to skillet and cook until heated through, for about 2 to 4 more minutes.

- Divide fajita mixture evenly onto tortillas.

- Serve immediately and enjoy.

NOTE:

When stored in the refrigerator in an air-tight container, this recipe can easily last up to 4-6 days, which makes chicken a great choice for your meal prep.

PREP TIME: 10 mins

COOK TIME: 15 mins

TOTAL TIME: 25 mins

YIELD: 4 servings

VEGGIE RICE

Rice is high in carbohydrates, but some types of rice like brown rice, are a whole grain food.

This kind of Veggie Rice is extremely high in carbs because it's loaded with veggies. Adding vegetables not only enhances its vitamin value but also contributes lots of fiber that prevents a quick rise in blood sugar levels after a meal.

INGREDIENTS

- 4 tablespoons of oil
- 2 cups of water
- 1 cup of basmati rice
- 1 small onion finely chopped
- 1/2 cup of frozen veggies. You can use a mix of corn, carrots, peas and green beans
- Salt and pepper to taste.

PREPARATIONS

- Heat the oil in a pot and fry the onion till translucent.
- Add the pepper, frozen veggies, salt and cook for 5 minutes.
- Add the water, and use lid to cover the pot.
- Bring water to a boil and then add the rice.
- Cook on medium high heat till rice is almost cooked and most of the water has evaporated.
- Lower the heat and cover the rice.

- Let the rice steam until it's completely cooked, for about 5 minutes.

- Remove from heat and use fork to fluff the rice.

- Serve immediately.

- Enjoy.

NOTE:

To preserve veggie rice, it is best to freeze it as soon as possible after cooking. Pack the veggie rice into a microwavable container as soon as it is cooked. When cooled, seal the container and place into the freezer. You can keep rice in the freezer for up to one month and it will still retain its moisture and taste, but you shouldn't leave it in the freezer much longer than that.

PREP TIME: 5 mins

COOK TIME: 20 mins

TOTAL TIME: 25 mins

YIELD: 4 servings

GRILLED TUNA KEBABS

Try Grilled Tuna Kebabs when you're looking to cook out. It's packed with fresh herbs and lime juice that brighten these skewers of tuna.

Enjoy the warm weather with this healthy grilled tuna kebabs recipe. They are a smart choice if you follow a diabetic diet, and so delicious enough for the whole family.

INGREDIENTS

- 3 tablespoons of fresh lime juice (from 2 limes)
- freshly ground pepper and coarse salt.
- 1 1/2 pounds of sushi-grade yellowfin tuna (cut into 1 1/2-inch cubes)
- 1/4 cup plus 2 tablespoons of extra-virgin olive oil
- 3 tablespoons of chopped fresh cilantro

PREPARATIONS

- Heat a grill pan over medium heat.
- Toss tuna with 1 tablespoon of oil.
- Thread tuna onto 4 kebabs.
- Combine lime juice, cilantro and 1/4 cup of oil.
- Season with pepper and salt.
- Reserve about 3 tablespoons.
- Brush pan with the remaining tablespoon of oil.

- Grill tuna, turning kebabs and brushing tuna occasionally with lime sauce, for about 2 minutes per side for rare or to desired doneness.

- Transfer kebabs to a serving plate.

- Brush with reserved lime sauce.

- Serve immediately and enjoy.

NOTE:

If it has been sitting out for more than two hours at room temperature, toss it. On a hotter day (above 90 degrees Fahrenheit), make that one hour. If you haven't exceeded the time limit, then place it in a shallow pan being careful not to over pack it. Cover and place near the top of the refrigerator. Eat within a few days or toss.

PREP TIME: 15 mins

COOK TIME: 0 mins

TOTAL TIME: 20 mins

YIELD: 4 servings

SPICY TURKEY TACOS

Tacos can be tasty and permissible in your diet. Add as many veggies you can to top it. It is a very versatile recipe that uses ground turkey to lower calories. It also makes for light and healthy tacos, simple and plain.

This Tacos recipe is also easy to prepare, healthy and delicious at the same time. Are you looking for Dinner recipe that is full of flavor? then this is the right recipe for you. Try it and you would be wowed!

INGREDIENTS

- 1/2 teaspoon of ground cumin
- 2 cups of shredded lettuce
- 8 taco shells
- 1/2 teaspoon of dried oregano
- 1/2 teaspoon of paprika
- 1/2 teaspoon of ground cinnamon
- 1 pound of extra-lean ground turkey
- 1 small red onion, finely chopped
- 1 cup of salsa
- 1/2 cup of shredded pepper jack cheese
- 1/4 cup of fat-free sour cream
- Cubed avocado and extra salsa, optional

PREPARATIONS

- Heat taco shells just according to the directions in the package.

- Cook turkey and onion in a large nonstick skillet over medium heat until the meat is no longer pink.

- Stir in spices and salsa.

- Heat through and serve immediately.

- Fill each of the taco shell with 1/3 cup of turkey mixture if you want to serve.

- Serve with cheese, lettuce or sour cream if you feel like.

- Enjoy.

NOTE:

To preserve this lovely recipe, cool completely and then measure into Ziploc freezer bags. Be sure to remove all of the air from the bag before sealing. Label the bag and the amount of Taco Meat you put into the bag. To thaw it, just pull it out of the freezer and let it thaw overnight in the fridge. Or you can run the bag under cold water until it is loosened up enough to dump out of the bag. Heat on the stovetop or in the microwave and use.

PREP TIME: 15 mins

COOK TIME: 0 mins

TOTAL TIME: 25 mins

YIELD: 4 servings

LIME QUINOA WITH CILANTRO

Quinoa has more protein than any other grain. This is a refreshing recipe that tastes good and makes up for a filling dinner as well. Apart from being very nutritious, quinoa has a very low glycemic index and gluten free which helps in keeping blood sugar under control.

The good news about this recipe is it even helps in reducing weight and it's full of refreshing flavor.

INGREDIENTS

- 1 mango, diced and peeled
- 1 diced jalapeno pepper
- 1/4 teaspoon of salt
- 1 avocado - peeled, pitted, and diced
- 1 1/2 tablespoons of lime juice
- 2 tablespoons of chopped fresh cilantro
- 1 tablespoon of olive oil
- 2 cloves garlic, minced
- 1/2 red onion, diced
- 1 cup of quinoa, rinsed and drained
- 1 1/2 cups of low-sodium chicken broth
- 1 cup of corn

PREPARATIONS

- In a saucepan, heat olive oil over medium heat

- Cook and stir garlic until fragrant for about 1 minute.

- Add jalapeno pepper, onion and salt.

- Cook and stir for about 5 to 10 minutes, until onion is tender.

- Add quinoa and cook for 2 minutes until slightly browned.

- Pour in the chicken broth, then bring to a boil.

- Reduce heat to low and simmer for about 15 minutes until broth is absorbed.

- Stir mango, corn, lime juice, avocado and cilantro into the quinoa mixture.

- Serve immediately and enjoy.

NOTE:

Consider freezing the leftovers for an easy side for future meals. Just let the quinoa cool completely before freezing.

PREP TIME: 20 mins

COOK TIME: 25 mins

TOTAL TIME: 45 mins

YIELD: 6 servings

POTATOES WITH ROASTED VEGGIES

MY **BONUS** RECIPE

Do you know you can have a healthy serving of roasted veggies with potatoes? This recipe is loaded with veggies that is so easy to prepare. It can be made a day ahead. What you have to do the next day is just 'reheat' before serving. You can use lemon juice if you don't have balsamic vinegar on hand. By the way, people with diabetes should be mindful of the portions of potato they consume. It shouldn't be too much.

INGREDIENTS

- 1 red onion, quartered
- 1 tablespoon of chopped fresh thyme
- 2 tablespoons of chopped fresh rosemary
- 1/4 cup of olive oil
- 2 tablespoons of balsamic vinegar
- 1 small butternut squash, cubed
- 2 red bell peppers, deseeded and diced
- 1 sweet potato, peeled and cubed
- 3 Yukon Gold potatoes, cubed
- salt and freshly ground black pepper

74

PREPARATIONS

- Preheat oven to 475 degrees F.

- Combine the red bell peppers, squash, Yukon gold potatoes and sweet potato in a large bowl.

- Separate the red onion quarters into pieces, then add them into the mixture.

- Stir together rosemary, thyme, vinegar, salt, olive oil, pepper and salt in a small bowl.

- Toss with vegetables till they're coated.

- Spread evenly on a large roasting pan.

- Roast for about 35 minutes in the preheated oven, until vegetables are cooked through and browned, turn the vegetables every 10 minutes.

- Serve and enjoy.

NOTE:

Refrigerate the potatoes in shallow airtight containers or resealable plastic bags. Properly stored, cooked potatoes with roasted veggies will last for 3 to 5 days in the refrigerator.

PREP TIME: 15 mins

COOK TIME: 40 mins

TOTAL TIME: 55 mins

YIELD: 12 servings

MUSHROOM STROGANOFF

MY **BONUS** RECIPE

The picture may not look appetizing but it's just so good. This is a diabetic recipe that is so rich, thick and can be eaten for dinner.

This recipe makes a great meal for diabetics as they contain very low amount of carbs, which means they don't raise blood sugar levels. They also have a very low glycaemic index.

INGREDIENTS

- 3 cloves garlic, minced
- 4 teaspoons of chopped fresh thyme
- 2 1/2 tablespoons of all-purpose flour
- 2 cups of beef stock
- 2 tablespoons of chopped fresh parsley leaves
- 8 ounces of medium pasta shells
- 3 tablespoons of unsalted butter
- 1 1/2 pounds of cremini mushrooms, thinly sliced
- 2 large shallots, diced
- Kosher salt and freshly ground black pepper, to taste
- 1 1/2 teaspoons of Dijon mustard
- 3/4 cup of sour cream
- 2/3 cup of freshly grated Parmesan

PREPARATIONS

- Cook pasta according to package instructions in a large pot of boiling salted water. Drain it well.

- In a large skillet, melt butter over medium high heat.

- Add shallots and mushrooms and cook, stirring occasionally, until mushrooms are browned and tender, for about 5 minutes.

- Season with pepper and salt, to taste.

- Stir in thyme and garlic, cook for 1 minute, until fragrant.

- Whisk in flour cook for 1 minute, until lightly browned.

- Whisk in beef stock and Dijon gradually and bring it to a boil.

- Reduce heat and simmer, stirring occasionally, until slightly thickened and reduced, for about 5 minutes.

- Stir in sour cream and pasta until heated through, for about 2 minutes.

- Stir in Parmesan for 1 minute, until melted.

- Stir in parsley, season with pepper and salt, to taste.

- Serve immediately and enjoy.

NOTE:

This vegan mushroom stroganoff sauce keeps in the refrigerator for 2 to 3 days or can be frozen for up to 2 months. I recommend storing or freeze the sauce separately from the pasta in a sealed container. When ready to serve, defrost overnight in the fridge, then heat it up on the stovetop and serve with your favorite side and fresh herbs.

PREP TIME: 10 mins

COOK TIME: 20 mins

TOTAL TIME: 30 mins

YIELD : 4 servings

DESSERT RECIPES

SUGAR FREE BUCKEYE BALLS

These delicious tasting Sugar Free Buckeye Balls are the perfect treat to share with your families and friends. They are low in carbs and diabetic friendly, because it's made with zero sugar.

We'll be adding a Sugar Free Peanut butter to this recipe. They actually work together in creating delicious taste.

INGREDIENTS

- 6 cups of Sugar Free Powdered Sugar

- 1 teaspoon of Vanilla Extract

- 1 1/2 cups of Sugar Free Peanut Butter

- 1 cup of Butter very soft

- 4 cups of Sugar Free Chocolate Chips

PREPARATIONS

- Prepare a baking sheet with wax paper. Set it aside.

- Cream together the sugar-free peanut butter, vanilla extract and sugar free powdered sugar in a mixing bowl.

- Form the mixture into 1 - 1 1/2-inches balls by rolling the dough in your hands.

- Place each of the ball on the wax prepared baking sheet.

- Place the prepared balls into the freezer for about 25 minutes, until hard.

- Melt the chocolate in a microwave when you're ready to dip the balls in the chocolate or using the double boiler method.

- Stir well as the chocolate melts.

- Remove the peanut butter balls from the freezer and dip each of it into the chocolate. You can leave the area around where you put your toothpick.

- Then place each ball back onto the wax paper and refrigerate them.

- Melt more if you run low on chocolate.

- Serve and enjoy.

NOTE:

The buckeye balls should be stored in an airtight container in the refrigerator to keep them nice and fresh. Stored in this way, they will keep for about 1 month. You can also freeze buckeyes in an airtight container or freezer Ziploc bag for up to 3 months.

PREP TIME: 20 mins

FREEZING TIME: 35 mins

TOTAL TIME: 55 mins

YIELD : 36 balls

PEANUT BUTTER COOKIES

I believe a healthy diet should absolutely include dessert. So if you're looking for the best cookie to enjoy, this Peanut Butter cookies are a healthy way to satisfy your cookie craving after having your breakfast or lunch meal.

They taste good and they come together in a bowl with just 2 ingredients for a super treat.

INGREDIENTS

- 1/2 teaspoon of baking soda
- 1/2 teaspoon of vanilla essence
- 1 cup of smooth peanut butter (no added sugar)
- 1 large egg
- 2/3 cup of erythritol

PREPARATIONS

- Preheat oven to 350 degrees F.
- Line a cookie tray with baking paper and set it aside.
- Add the erythritol to a blender and blend until powdered. Set it aside. (Skip this step if using a confectioner's low carb sweetener).
- In a medium mixing bowl, add all of the ingredients and mix until smooth and glossy dough forms.
- Roll about 2 tablespoons of dough in your palms to form a ball, and place on the prepared cookie tray. Repeat until you consume the doughs. You will end up with 12 to 14 cookies.
- Use a fork to flatten the cookies and create a criss cross patten across the top.

- Bake the cookies for about 12 minutes.

- Remove from the oven and allow it to cool on the baking tray, for about 25 minutes.

- Transfer into a cooling rack for another 15 minutes.

- Serve and enjoy.

NOTE:

At room temperature, you can store these cookies in an airtight container for up to 4 to 6 days (they will last past that point, they just won't be as good). In the freezer, these cookies can be frozen in an airtight container or freezer bag up to 3 months.

PREP TIME: 5 mins

COOK TIME: 15 mins

COOLING TIME: 40 mins

TOTAL TIME: 1 hour

YIELD: 12 balls

CHOCOLATE FUDGE

MY **BONUS** RECIPE

Chocolate Fudge is a simple recipe you can make. It's vegan, low carb, keto and even diabetic friendly.

It can be ready to eat with just 3 to 5 simple ingredients. You just have to let it set very well in the fridge for some hours. I hope you enjoy it!

INGREDIENTS

- 10 ounces of bittersweet chocolate chips
- *Optional:* coarse or flaked sea salt for topping
- 1 1/2 cups of coconut butter
- 1 (13.66 FL ounces) can of full-fat coconut milk

PREPARATIONS

- Use paper or foil to line an 8 by 8 inch baking pan.
- Melt the coconut butter in a small saucepan over low heat.
- Stir in the chocolate chips and coconut milk.
- Cook over low heat, stirring consistently, until the chocolate chips are melted.
- Pour the mixture into the pan.
- Place in refrigerator for about 2 hours, until set.
- Slice, serve and enjoy.

NOTE:

Place the wrapped chocolate fudge inside an airtight container for additional protection from moisture loss, which may cause fudge to become dry and crumbly. Store at room temperature for two to three weeks. Transfer it to the refrigerator if you plan to store it for longer.

PREP TIME: 5 mins

COOK TIME: 2 hours

TOTAL TIME: 2 hours 5 mins

YIELD: 40 squares

LOW-CARB CHEESECAKE

MY **BONUS** RECIPE

This is a healthy low carb cheesecake that is simply delicious and so simple to make. This recipe would definitely satisfy your cheesecake cravings.

This dessert is so healthy that you can eat it as a snack whenever you feel like without feeling guilty at all. It's just so perfect. A perfect recipe for a mid-morning snack or after your workout (before morning meal.)

INGREDIENTS

- 1 tablespoon of Stevia
- 1 teaspoon of vanilla extract
- 8.5 ounces of low fat cottage cheese
- 2 egg whites
- 1 scoop of vanilla protein powder
- 1 serving sugar-free Strawberry Jell-O
- Water

PREPARATIONS

- Preheat the oven to 325 degrees F.
- Prepare the Jell-O according to the instructions on the package.
- Place in the freezer.

- Blend egg whites and cottage cheese until the consistency is smooth.

- Pour the blended mixture inside the bowl.

- Whisk it together with the stevia, protein powder and vanilla extract.

- Transfer the batter into a small nonstick pan, then bake for about 25 minutes.

- Turn off the oven (but let the cake in it cool down).

- Remove the cheesecake once the oven has cooled.

- Pour it over the cheesecake when the Jell-O is almost set.

- Let the cake set in the fridge for about 10 hours before enjoying.

- Now you can serve and enjoy.

NOTE:

Simply slice the pieces of cheesecake and place them on individual pieces of plastic wrap. Wrap them tight, place in a freezer bag or bowl, and store them in the freezer for up to 2 weeks. Any longer than 2 weeks and they will lose quality.

PREP TIME: 10 mins

COOK TIME: 50 mins

TOTAL TIME: 1 hour

YIELD: 2 servings

30 DAYS DIABETIC MEAL PLAN FOR BEGINNERS

DIABETIC MEAL PLAN (DAYS 1 - 7)

DAY	BREAKFAST	LUNCH	DINNER
1	Mini Veggie Quiche	Chicken Tortilla Soup	French Lentils
2	Shakshuka	Leftover Chicken Tortilla Soup	Leftover French Lentils
3	Leftover Shakshuka	Chicken Broccoli Salad	Veggie Rice
4	Healthy Granola	Black Bean Salad	Chicken Fajitas
5	Leftover Healthy Granola	Leftover Chicken Tortilla Soup	Leftover Veggie Rice
6	Cinnamon Oat Muffins with Apple	Leftover Black Bean Salad	Leftover Chicken Fajitas
7	Leftover Healthy Granola	Chicken Broccoli Salad	Leftover French Lentils

DIABETIC MEAL PLAN (DAYS 8 - 14)

DAY	BREAKFAST	LUNCH	DINNER
8	Veggie Frittata	Kale Salad with Lemon Dressing	Grilled Tuna Kebabs
9	Veggie Omelet	Carrot Ginger Soup	Spicy Turkey Tacos
10	Leftover Veggie Frittata	Leftover Kale Salad with Lemon Dressing	Leftover Grilled Tuna Kebabs
11	Egg Pepper Cups	Shrimp Salad	Lime Quinoa with Cilantro
12	Leftover Egg Pepper Cups	Leftover Carrot Ginger Soup	Leftover Lime Quinoa with Cilantro
13	Leftover Egg Pepper Cups	Leftover Kale Salad with Lemon Dressing	Mushroom Stroganoff
14	Leftover Veggie Omelet	Leftover Shrimp Salad	Leftover Mushroom Stroganoff

DIABETIC MEAL PLAN (DAYS 15 - 21)

DAY	BREAKFAST	LUNCH	DINNER
15	Cinnamon Oat Muffins With Apple	Crispy Tofu	Potatoes with Roasted Veggies
16	Leftover Cinnamon Oat Muffins With Apple	Spinach Soup with Pesto & Chicken	Leftover Potatoes with Roasted Veggies
17	Coconut Porridge	Leftover Crispy Tofu	French Lentils
18	Mini Veggie Quiche	Tortilla Chicken Soup	Veggie Rice
19	Leftover Coconut Porridge	Chicken Broccoli Salad	Leftover French Lentils
20	Leftover Cinnamon Oat Muffins With Apple	Black Bean Salad	Leftover Veggie Rice
21	Leftover Coconut Porridge	Kale Salad With Lemon Dressing	Leftover Veggie Rice

DIABETIC MEAL PLAN (DAYS 22 - 30)

DAY	BREAKFAST	LUNCH	DINNER
22	Healthy Granola	Tortilla Chicken Soup	Potatoes with Roasted Veggies
23	Veggie Omelet	Leftover Tortilla Chicken Soup	French Lentils
24	Shakshuka	Kale Salad With Lemon Dressing	Leftover Potatoes with Roasted Veggies
25	Mini Veggie Quiche	Black Bean Salad	Chicken Fajitas
26	Leftover Veggie Omelet	Carrot Ginger Soup	Leftover French Lentils
27	Leftover Mini Veggie Quiche	Shrimp Salad	Veggie Rice
28	Leftover Shakshuka	Leftover Carrot Ginger Soup	Grilled Tuna Kebabs
29	Veggie Frittata	Leftover Shrimp Salad	Leftover Veggie Rice
30	Leftover Veggie Frittata	Crispy Tofu	Leftover Grilled Tuna Kebabs

THANK YOU!
DIABETIC MEAL PREP
FOR BEGINNERS

Table Of Contents

50 EASY DIABETIC DESSERT RECIPES
by STELLA WATERS

Do you miss being able to eat something sweet every once and awhile?

A diabetes diagnoses usually means that you can no longer eat sweets or other sugary desserts ever again. This book is filled with all sorts of cakes, brownies and other delicious desserts that will have you looking forward to staying on your diabetic diet.

This book contains everything that you have a missed eating, now back with diabetic safe recipes, so you can enjoy them just like you used too. And best of all, your family can too; these sweet and savory desserts are so good that most people can't tell the difference. Best of all, no matter the celebration, holiday or family event, you will be able to bring a delicious, diabetic safe dessert.

If you are tired of eating the same old diabetic diets, then you need this book. Filled with tons of family favorite recipes which have been reworked to taste great and be diabetic safe. Unlike other books, these recipes are all about taste, if it does not taste great then it is not in the book.

The reason for this is that great recipes are meant to be shared with those closest to you, whether they are diabetic or not. That way, you and your family can eat cake and share cookies together, just like you used to.

What's in this book?

- ➢ Muffins
- ➢ Cakes
- ➢ Cookies
- ➢ Sweet Fat-Bombs
- ➢ Desserts
- ➢ Snacks and Treats
- ➢ Diabetic Fruity Desserts

- **Diabetic Safe Pies:**
Everything from Apple Pie to Lemon Cream Pie all made so you can eat it without worries.

- **Diabetic Safe Cakes and Brownies:**
From Carrot Cakes to Chocolate Brownies, these recipes are so good that diabetics and non-diabetics both can enjoy it.

- **Diabetic Safe Cookies:**
From Banana Cookies to Gingersnap's, this book has enough cookie recipes to keep you and your family happy for years.

Thanks for choosing this book, make sure to **leave a short review** on Amazon if you enjoy it. I'd really love to hear your thoughts

Enjoy! ☺

Stella Waters.

EASY
DIABETIC
DESSERT
RECIPES

CHOCO FAT BOMBS

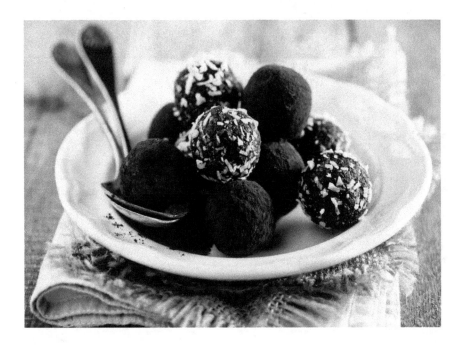

Choco Fat Bombs is a great recipe to increase your fat intake and help satisfy your chocolate cravings. If you need a savory diabetic dessert recipe, this Fat Bomb is the right recipe to have.

I highly recommend trying this dessert. It's packed with awesome flavor and it's incredibly easy. To make this recipe, all you need is your fridge or freezer, a bowl, and a tray with parchment paper.

INGREDIENTS

- 2 tablespoons of heavy cream
- 1 teaspoon of vanilla extract
- 2 tablespoons of Stevia
- 1/4 cup of unsweetened cocoa powder
- 5 tablespoons of natural chunky peanut butter
- 6 tablespoons of hemp seeds (shelled)
- 1/2 cup of unrefined coconut oil

PREPARATIONS

- Mix peanut butter, cocoa powder, and hemp seeds in a large bowl.
- Add room temperature coconut oil and mix till it becomes a paste.
- Add vanilla, cream, and stevia. Mix until it becomes a paste again.
- Roll into balls. When rolling, you should make up to 12 balls in total.
- Put in the fridge, if the paste is too thin to roll, for about 30 minutes before rolling.
- Roll in shredded coconut.
- Place balls on parchment paper on a baking tray.
- Put in the fridge for at least 30 minutes before serving.
- Serve and enjoy.
- Store the leftover in the fridge.

PREP TIME : 15 mins
FREEZE TIME : 10 mins
TOTAL TIME : 25 mins
YIELD : 12 balls

LOW-CARB CHEESECAKE

This healthy Low Carb Cheesecake is a simple and delicious recipe to make. This cheesecake recipe is the right answer to your cravings. It helps satisfy your cheesecake cravings without blowing a whole week's calorie budget.

For a cake with almost no fat, calories, or carbs, it tastes absolutely amazing. You'll always get high praise when you serve it to your health-conscious families and friends.

They will love it. I promise!

INGREDIENTS

- 1 tablespoon of stevia
- 1 teaspoon of vanilla extract
- 1 serving of sugar-free Strawberry Jell-O
- 8.5 ounces of low-fat cottage cheese
- 2 egg whites
- 1 scoop vanilla protein powder
- Water

PREPARATIONS

- Preheat the oven to 325 degrees F.
- Prepare the Jell-O according to the package directions.
- Place in the freezer.
- Blend egg whites and cottage cheese until the consistency is smooth.
- In a bowl, pour the blended mixture, and whisk it together with the stevia, protein powder, and vanilla extract.
- In a small nonstick pan, transfer the batter. Bake for about 25 minutes.
- Turn off the oven.
- Leave the cake in the oven while it cools down.
- Remove the cheesecake from the oven once it has cooled.
- Pour it over the cheesecake when the Jell-O is almost set (you should be able to stir it).
- Let the cake set in the fridge before serving, for about 10 hours minimum.
- Serve and enjoy.

PREP TIME : 10 mins
COOK TIME : 50 mins
TOTAL TIME : 1 hour
YIELD : 2 servings

PROTEIN BUTTER COOKIES

I believe a healthy diabetic diet should absolutely include dessert. So, if you're looking for the best cookies to enjoy, these Peanut Butter Cookies are a healthy way to satisfy your cookie craving after having your breakfast or lunch meal.

They taste good and they come together in a bowl with just five ingredients for a super treat.

INGREDIENTS

- 2/3 cup of erythritol
- 1/2 teaspoon of baking soda
- 1 cup of smooth peanut butter (no added sugar)
- 1 large egg
- 1/2 teaspoon of vanilla essence

PREPARATIONS

- Preheat oven to 350 degrees F.
- Use baking paper to line a cookie tray and set it aside.
- Add the erythritol into a blender or nutribullet.
- Blend until powdered and set it aside. You can skip this step if you'll be using a confectioner's low-carb sweetener.
- In a medium mixing bowl, add all of the ingredients and mix until a glossy smooth dough forms.
- Roll about 2 tablespoons of dough between your palms to form a ball.
- Then place on the prepared cookie tray.
- Repeat until all dough has been used. You should end up with 12 to 15 cookies.
- Flatten the cookies using a fork, creating a crisscross pattern across the top.
- Bake for about 12 to 15 minutes.
- Remove from the oven.
- Allow to cool on the baking tray, for about 25 minutes.
- Then transfer into a cooling rack for another 15 minutes.
- Serve and enjoy.

PREP TIME : 5 mins
COOK TIME : 15 mins
FREEZE TIME : 40 mins
TOTAL TIME : 1 hour
YIELD : 12 servings

RASPBERRY MUFFINS WITH PUMPKIN

Nobody will believe that this particular Raspberry Muffins with Pumpkin recipe is actually low-fat, low-carb, sugar-free, and diabetic friendly. They won't believe it until you tell them.

They are very simple to put together, and also, they will become a family favorite for either breakfast, lunch boxes, or snacks. This dessert recipe can be shared at parties and you would have fun watching people eating them and praising you.

INGREDIENTS

- 1 cup of pumpkin puree - canned
- 1/2 cup of coconut flour
- 3/4 cup of blanched almond flour
- 1/2 cup of Stevia
- 1/4 teaspoon of salt
- 4 (1/2 cup) egg whites
- 4 egg yolks
- 1/2 cup of coconut oil (melted)
- 1 1/2 teaspoon of vanilla extract
- 1 1/2 cup of frozen raspberries
- 10 drops of liquid stevia
- 3 tablespoons of arrowroot starch or tapioca
- 1 tablespoon of baking powder
- 1 tablespoon of cinnamon
- Pinch nutmeg

PREPARATIONS

- Preheat your oven to 350 degrees F.
- Use muffin papers to line 12 muffin cups.
- Stir together the almond flour, coconut flour, tapioca starch, stevia, cinnamon, baking powder, sea salt, and nutmeg in a large bowl until it is all mixed well.
- Stir in the pumpkin puree, stevia drops, coconut oil, vanilla and egg yolks (keep the egg whites separate for the next step) until completely incorporated.
- Beat the egg whites in a separate bowl until stiff white peaks form.
- Fold the frozen raspberries and egg whites into the muffin batter.
- At this stage, make sure to not mix the batter too much as the muffins will become denser if you do.
- Fold the egg whites and raspberries gently into the batter, using spatula or a spoon.
- Spoon the muffin batter into the muffin papers.
- Smooth out the tops.
- The batter should just be at the top of the muffin papers.
- Keep the muffin papers fuller to compensate as the muffins don't rise very high.
- Bake muffins for about 25 minutes.
- On the top of the muffins, it will be a light golden. Also, the toothpick should come out clean when inserted.
- Allow it to cool for about 5 minutes in the muffin tray before placing the muffins on a cooling rack to cool completely.
- Serve and enjoy.

PREP TIME : 10 mins
COOK TIME : 25 mins
COOL TIME : 20 mins
TOTAL TIME : 1 hour
YIELD : 12 muffins

STRAWBERRY POPSICLES WITH LEMON

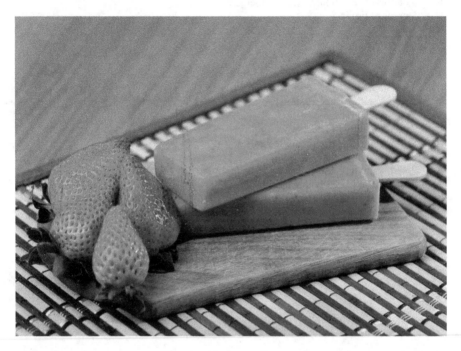

These healthy Strawberry Popsicles with Lemon have all the delicious flavors of a summer treat with zero sugar added. And with just five ingredients, your dessert will be ready to consume.

What makes this recipe unique are the old-fashioned oats and low-fat cottage cheese. Although, strawberries, stevia extract, and lemon juice are ingredients you would expect. I hope you love it, seriously.

They are a treat that anyone can feel good about eating, especially for people with diabetes like me.

INGREDIENTS

- 4 ounces of low-fat cottage cheese
- 1 and half pound of strawberries
- 1/4 cup of old-fashioned oats
- 4 ounces of lemon juice, (about 4 lemons)
- 5 drops of liquid Stevia

PREPARATIONS

- In a high powdered food processor or blender, pulse the oats until they turn into powder.
- Add the cottage cheese, strawberries, stevia and lemon juice.
- Then pulse until smooth.
- Stop the blender if necessary.
- Use a spatula to push the ingredients down.
- Do not add any liquid.
- Pour the mixture into your 6 Popsicle molds.
- Freeze for at least 3 hours, until solid.
- Serve and enjoy.

PREP TIME : 5 mins
FREEZE TIME : 3 hours
TOTAL TIME : 3 hours 5 mins
YIELD : 6 servings

KETO CHOCO FUDGE

This Keto Choco Fudge is so simple and it just happens to be keto, vegan, low carb, and diabetic-friendly.

This recipe is so dangerously easy, it takes just three simple ingredients and five minutes to be ready to eat. You just have to let it sit in the fridge for some hours. You know what I mean, right? You'll love it that way.

The result is creamy, smooth, and rich. I hope you love it.

Enjoy.

INGREDIENTS

- 10 ounces of bittersweet chocolate chips
- 1 1/2 cups of coconut butter
- 1 (13.66 FL ounces) can of full-fat coconut milk
- Optional: coarse or flaked sea salt for topping

PREPARATIONS

- Use foil or wax paper to line an 8 by 8-inch baking pan.
- Melt the coconut butter over low heat in a small saucepan.
- Stir in the chocolate chips and coconut milk.
- Cook over low heat, until the chocolate chips are melted.
- Stir frequently when cooking.
- Pour the mixture in a pan.
- Optional: Sprinkle coarse or flaked sea salt over the top.
- Place in the refrigerator for about 2 hours, until set.
- Slice and enjoy.

PREP TIME : 5 mins
CHILL TIME : 2 hours
TOTAL TIME : 2 hours 5 mins
YIELD : 40 squares

BANANA COOKIES

You don't need to change anything whatsoever in this recipe at all. The cookies tasted a bit like banana bread because of the cinnamon. This recipe will definitely rival yours. It's a great recipe you need to try today.

They are quite filling and make a great snack in the middle of the day. Do you know what I love about this recipe? My dear, you can get addicted to them. Lol.

I hope you love it.

INGREDIENTS

- 1 cup of raisins
- 1/3 cup of plain yogurt
- 3 very ripe bananas
- 2 cups of rolled oats
- 1 teaspoon of ground cinnamon

PREPARATIONS

- Preheat the oven to 350 degrees F.
- Use parchment paper to line cookie sheets.
- In a large bowl, mash bananas.
- Add raisins, yogurt, oats and cinnamon.
- Mix well.
- Allow it to sit for 15 minutes.
- Drop spoonful's of dough 2 inches apart onto the prepared cookie sheets.
- Bake in the preheated oven for about 20 minutes, until browned lightly.
- Serve and enjoy.

PREP TIME : 10 mins
CHILL TIME : 20 mins
ADDITIONAL TIME : 15 mins
TOTAL TIME : 45 mins
YIELD : 12 cookies

STRAWBERRY GRANITA

You can make this dessert recipe and serve anytime. But it is best enjoyed during the summer periods. It's extremely delicious and creamy, but heavy. This recipe is a great way to use an abundance of strawberries from your garden patch. Please make sure you eat this as a summer refresher :)

It's very simple and make sure to leave enough time for the freezing and stirring. You can make it in the morning and it will be ready to consume in the summer evenings.

Please make sure you don't omit the balsamic vinegar. This is because it adds brightness to the dish.

INGREDIENTS

- 1 cup of water
- 1/2 teaspoon of lemon juice (optional)
- 1/4 teaspoon of balsamic vinegar (optional)
- 2 pounds of ripe strawberries, halved and hulled
- 1/3 cup of white sugar, or to taste
- 1 tiny pinch of salt

PREPARATIONS

- Use cold water to rinse the strawberries.
- Transfer the berries into a blender.
- Add water, sugar, lemon juice, salt, and balsamic vinegar.
- To get the mixture moving, you need to pulse several times.
- Blend for about 1 minute, until smooth.
- Pour into a large baking dish (in the dish, the puree should be about 3/8 inch deep).
- In the freezer, place dish uncovered until mixture barely starts to freeze for about 45 minutes, around the edges.
- Mixture will still be slushy in the center.
- Stir the crystals from the edge of the granita mixture lightly into the center and mix thoroughly using a fork.
- Close freezer and chill for about 30 to 40 minutes, until granita is nearly frozen.
- Lightly mix with a fork before scraping the crystals loose.
- Repeat with freezing and stirring with fork until the granita is light, looks fluffy and dry, crystals are separate, for 3 to 4 times.
- Portion the granita into small serving bowls.
- Serve and enjoy.

PREP TIME : 10 mins
FREEZING TIME : 2 hours 10 mins
TOTAL TIME : 2 hours 25 mins
YIELD : 8 servings

BAKED APPLES

This easy Baked Apple recipe makes a great snack and/or dessert. You can use whatever fruit-flavored diet soda that catches your fancy.

This recipe is great with the diet orange. You can use diet Crush. You would smell the orange by the time you open the oven. Whipping with cream or strawberry yogurt on top is also a great way to enjoy this recipe.

INGREDIENTS

- 2 cups of sugar-free diet orange-flavored carbonated beverage
- 6 small apples, halved and cored

PREPARATIONS

- Preheat an oven to 350 degrees F.
- Arrange the apples into a baking dish with the cut sides facing down.
- Over the apples, pour the orange beverage.
- Bake in the preheated oven for about 1 hour, or until the apples are tender.
- Serve and enjoy.

PREP TIME : 5 mins
COOK TIME : 1 hour
TOTAL TIME : 1 hour 5 mins
YIELD : 6 servings

BANANA CHIA PUDDING

Banana Chia Pudding is the kind of diabetic dessert that is so easy to make, is delicious, and all-around awesome. You can use vanilla soy milk instead and making this recipe on a fairly regular basis would be great.

You'll never regret it. It's a fantastic snack with so many health benefits. It's awesome and delish.

Enjoy.

INGREDIENTS

- 3 tablespoons of honey
- 1 teaspoon of vanilla extract
- 1/8 teaspoon of sea salt
- 1 and 1/2 cups of vanilla-flavored flax milk
- 1 large banana, cut in chunks
- 7 tablespoons of Chai seeds

PREPARATIONS

- In the blender, put these in respective order: milk, banana, chia seeds, honey, vanilla extract, and sea salt.
- Blend together until smooth.
- Pour mixture into a bowl.
- Refrigerate for at least 2 hours, until thickened.
- Spoon mixture into small bowls to serve.
- Serve and enjoy.

PREP TIME : 10 mins
COOK TIME : 2 hours
TOTAL TIME : 2 hours 10 mins
YIELD : 6 servings

MEXICAN MANGO

If you want to enjoy this Mexican Mango, you can make it in the morning, cool it and put it in the refrigerator. Then at dinner, heat it for a couple of seconds in the microwave. In fact, you can just double the recipe. You'll definitely add it to your favorites.

You can serve with coconut shrimp and steak. So nice and delicious.

INGREDIENTS

- 1 pinch of salt
- 3 tablespoons of lemon juice
- 1/4 cup of water
- 1 tablespoon of chili powder
- 1 mango - seeded, peeled, and sliced

PREPARATIONS

- In a small saucepan, bring water to a boil.
- Stir in salt, chili powder, and lemon juice until hot and smooth.
- Add sliced mango and toss to coat.
- Allow it to soak up the chili sauce for some minutes before serving.
- Serve and enjoy.

PREP TIME : 5 mins
COOK TIME : 10 mins
TOTAL TIME : 15 mins
YIELD : 2 servings

BANANA ICE CREAM

Please do not throw your banana away when they are overripe. All you need to do is peel them, wrap them in plastic wrap, and freeze them. Only two ingredients is all you need to make this family pleaser.

Enjoy.

INGREDIENTS

- 1/2 cup of skim milk
- 2 chopped and peeled bananas, frozen

PREPARATIONS

- Combine 1/4 cup of skim milk and frozen bananas in a blender.
- Blend for about 30 seconds.
- Add remaining 1/4 cup of milk.
- Blend for about 30 seconds on high speed until smooth.
- Serve and enjoy.

PREP TIME : 5 mins
COOK TIME : 0 mins
TOTAL TIME : 5 mins
YIELD : 2 servings

APPLE PIE

For this recipe, using apple juice is a great idea. When you use sugar substitutes, the pie will seem dry - that would help solve that problem.

Make this recipe for your family's thanksgiving feast. No one in the family group will even know this is a diabetic Apple Pie.

You can stick to your apple juice flavor. It'll give the pie a really nice added flavor. What I love about this recipe is that it will be great the next day.

INGREDIENTS

- 1/3 cup of thawed apple juice concentrate
- Pastry for double-crust pie (9 inches)
- 8 cups of thinly sliced peeled tart apples
- 1 tablespoon of butter
- Sugar substitute equivalent to 8 teaspoons of sugar
- 2 teaspoons of cornstarch
- 1 teaspoon of ground cinnamon

PREPARATIONS

- Combine the apple juice, sugar, cornstarch, and cinnamon together.
- Line a pie plate with a bottom crust; add apples.
- Over the apples, pour juice mixture and dot with butter.
- Roll out the rest of the pastry to the fit top of pie.
- Cut slits or an apple shape in top.
- Place over filling; flute and seal edges.
- Bake at 375 degrees for about 35 minutes.
- Increase heat to 400 degrees.
- Bake until apples are tender for about 15 to 20 minutes.
- Serve and enjoy.

PREP TIME : 15 mins
BAKE TIME : 50 mins
TOTAL TIME : 1 hour 5 mins
YIELD : 8 servings

GRILLED PEACHES

Grilled peaches are the kind of magic that happens in a hot grill's twilight, and it's the best pairing for the cold wine and ice cream destined for dessert.

The truth about these grilled peaches is that they are surprisingly simple, and they just require olive oil and fresh peaches to prepare on a cooling grill.

The finished peaches should not be falling apart with distinct grill marks and it should be more tender. Actually, most of the peach skin will be slipping away and you just need to pull these off using your tongs before serving if you feel like it. Enjoy.

INGREDIENTS

- 6 peaches (freestone)
- Olive oil

PREPARATIONS

Preparing the grill:

- Light a gas grill to medium heat.
- Grill the peaches after everything else has been grilled. That is if you'll be cooking over charcoal.

Making the grilled peaches:

- Halve the pit of peaches by running a sharp knife along each of the peach's seam to halve them.
- Remove the pit and use olive oil to brush each cut side.
- Place the peaches cut side down on the grill.
- Cook undisturbed for about 4 to 5 minutes, until grill marks appear.
- Flip the peaches, then grill for about 4 to 5 minutes more, until the peaches are soft and skins are charred.
- Remove from the grill.
- Serve the grilled peaches with butter or vanilla ice cream.
- Enjoy.

PREP TIME : 5 mins
COOK TIME : 10 mins
TOTAL TIME : 15 mins
YIELD : 8 servings

PEANUT BUTTER SWIRL BROWNIES

This diabetic-friendly brownie recipe uses the classic combination of peanut butter and chocolate to make a delicious dessert you will want to make again and again.

It's not too cakey and not too fudgy. But sincerely, you would love it.

Enjoy!

INGREDIENTS

- 1 teaspoon of vanilla
- 1 1/4 cups of whole-wheat pastry flour, divided
- 1 teaspoon of baking powder
- 1/4 cup of creamy peanut butter
- 1/2 cup of unsweetened cocoa powder
- Nonstick cooking spray
- 1/4 cup of butter
- 3/4 cup of granulated sugar
- 1/3 cup of cold water
- 3/4 cup of refrigerated or frozen egg product, thawed, or 3 eggs (lightly beaten)
- 1/4 cup of canola oil
- 1/4 cup of miniature semisweet chocolate pieces

PREPARATIONS

- Preheat the oven to 350 degrees F.
- Use foil to line a 9x9x2 inch baking pan, extend foil up over the edges of the pan.
- Use nonstick spray to lightly coat foil and set it aside.
- Melt butter in a medium saucepan over low heat.
- Remove from heat.
- Whisk in the water and sugar.
- Whisk in oil, egg, and vanilla until combined.
- Stir in the baking powder and 1 cup of the flour until combined.
- In a small bowl, place the peanut butter; gradually whisk in 1/2 cup of the batter until smooth and set it aside.
- Combine the cocoa powder and the rest 1/4 cup of flour in a separate bowl.
- Stir into the plain batter.
- Stir in chocolate pieces and pour the chocolate batter into the prepared pan.
- In small mounds, drop peanut butter batter over chocolate batter in pan.
- Swirl batter together using a thin metal spatula.
- Bake until a toothpick inserted in the center comes out clean and the top springs back when lightly touched, for about 20 to 25 minutes.
- Cool completely in a pan over a wire rack.
- Cut into bars.
- Serve and enjoy.

PREP TIME : 15 mins
COOK TIME : 0 mins
TOTAL TIME : 40 mins
YIELD : 20 servings

ALMOND QUINOA BLONDIES

More than likely, people won't even notice that these chocolaty, delicately nutty blondies are diabetic and gluten-free.

They use quinoa flour which you can find in natural food stores and well-stocked supermarkets, in the place of all-purpose flour. If you want to make your quinoa flour, you can grind raw quinoa into a powder using a clean coffee grinder.

You can use almond extract instead of vanilla. It will still add a lovely flavor to this dessert. Enjoy.

INGREDIENTS

- 1 teaspoon of vanilla extract
- 3/4 cup of quinoa flour
- 1 teaspoon of baking powder
- 1/4 teaspoon of salt
- 1/4 cup of unsalted butter, softened
- 3/4 cup of crunchy or smooth natural almond butter
- 2 large eggs
- 3/4 cup of packed light brown sugar
- 1 cup of semisweet chocolate chips

PREPARATIONS

- Preheat oven to 350 degrees F.
- Use parchment paper or foil to line an 8-inch square baking pan.
- Allow it to overhang opposite ends slightly.
- Use cooking spray to coat.
- Beat almond butter and butter in a bowl until creamy using an electric mixer.
- Beat in brown sugar, eggs and vanilla.
- Whisk baking powder, quinoa flour, and salt in a small bowl.
- Mix the flour mixture into the wet ingredients until just combined.
- Stir in chocolate chips.
- Evenly spread the butter into the prepared pan.
- Bake for about 25 to 35 minutes or until a toothpick inserted into the center comes out with just some little moist crumbs.
- Do not overbake it.
- Let it cool in the pan for about 45 minutes.
- Lift the whole pan out using the parchment or foil and transfer to a cutting board.
- Cut into squares and serve and enjoy.

PREP TIME : 15 mins
COOL TIME : 1 hour 20 mins
TOTAL TIME : 1 hour 35 mins
YIELD : 24 servings

FRUIT YOGURT POPSICLES

These popsicles have more strawberry than the yogurt. You can increase the amount of yogurt to 1 and a half cups if you would like closer to equal parts of strawberry and yogurt. Balancing the berries and yogurt will make you love this recipe.

These are not only great for snacks, but for dessert as well. I hope you enjoy it.

INGREDIENTS

For the simple syrup:
- 1/2 cup of water
- 1/2 cup of granulated sugar

For the Popsicles:
- 1 tablespoon of lemon juice
- 1 cup of plain or vanilla yogurt
- 1 pound (4 cups) of strawberries, halved and hulled

PREPARATIONS

- In a saucepan, stir the water and sugar together over medium heat.
- Bring to a boil and stir till the sugar dissolves.
- Chill until cold.
- Puree the strawberries, 3 tablespoons of the syrup and lemon juice in a food processor or blender until smooth.
- Taste and add more syrup if you feel like.
- Transfer into your measuring bowl or cup.
- Whisk the yogurt to smooth out the lumps in a bowl.
- Fill the molds by alternating 1 tablespoon of yogurt and 1 tablespoon of fruit.
- Continue alternating berries and yogurt until the molds are filled to 1/4-inch from the top.
- Poke deep into popsicle molds and swirl yogurt with fruit together using a chopstick or skewer.
- Freeze for an hour.
- Remove the mold from the freezer and insert the popsicle sticks inside, leaving about 2-inch of each stick above the mold.
- Return to the freezer until frozen, for another 3 hours.
- Dip the sides and bottom of the mold in a container of hot water and hold long enough to thaw the popsicles so they release from the mold.
- Serve and transfer into the store in the freezer.
- Enjoy.

PREP TIME : 10 mins
FREEZING TIME : 5 hours
TOTAL TIME : 5 hours 10 mins
YIELD : 10 popsicles

BAKED CINNAMON STUFFED IN APPLES

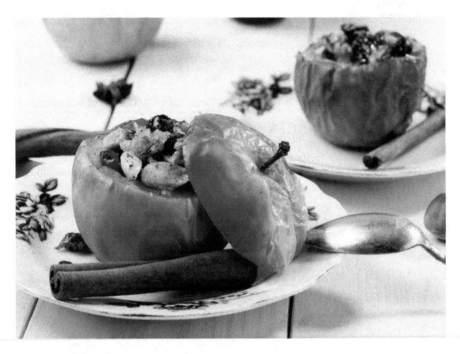

Yummy apples with oatmeal filling are a great way to enjoy your fall tree-picked apples.

Let me tell you something; this recipe is so delicious and perfect. A scoop of vanilla ice cream sends it over the top. You won't want to change this recipe because they are tender, juicy and can be ready within 30 minutes.

Your whole house will smell wonderful by the time you place the apples in the oven.

INGREDIENTS

- 4 apples
- 1 teaspoon of ground cinnamon
- 1/4 cup of butter
- 1 cup of rolled oats
- 1/4 cup of brown sugar

PREPARATIONS

- Preheat the oven to 350 degrees F.
- Core each of the apple.
- Make a large well in the center of each apple and arrange them on a rimmed baking sheet.
- Mix brown sugar, oats, and cinnamon together in a bowl.
- Cut in butter until evenly combined.
- Spoon 1/4 of the oat mixture into each apple.
- Bake in the preheated oven for about 30 minutes, or until apples are tender and filling is bubbling.
- Serve and enjoy.

PREP TIME : 15 mins
COOK TIME : 40 mins
TOTAL TIME : 45 mins
YIELD : 4 servings

DARK CHOCO ALMOND BARK

Dark Choco Almond Bark is a great treat for diabetics.

Adding sea salt to this treat would be great too. The combination of Dark Choco Almond Bark with sea salt will definitely satisfy your craving. And you would want to double your recipe because it doesn't last long.

Well, I hope you enjoy it too.

INGREDIENTS

- 1/8 teaspoon of sea salt
- 1/2 teaspoon of vanilla extract
- 1/4 cup of almonds chopped
- 1/8 teaspoon of sea salt optional
- 50 grams (about 1/2 cup) of cocoa butter
- 1/2 cup of unsweetened cocoa; you can use Ghirardelli
- 1/4 cup of low-carb sugar substitute or 1 tablespoon plus 2 teaspoons of Trivia
- 1/4 teaspoon of almonds finely chopped, optional

PREPARATIONS

- In a double boiler or chocolate melter, melt cocoa butter.
- Stir in sweetener, salt, and cocoa powder.
- Keep on heat until the dry ingredients have been incorporated very well into the melted cocoa butter.
- Remove from the heat.
- Stir in chopped almonds and vanilla extract.
- Pour out on a chocolate mold or prepared pan.
- Sprinkle with chopped almonds and additional salt if you want.
- Serve and enjoy.

PREP TIME : 5 mins
COOK TIME : 15 mins
TOTAL TIME : 20 mins
YIELD : 10 pieces

GINGER CUPCAKES

This Ginger Cupcake is one of my favorite holiday and diabetic recipes. It's warm and full of sweet spices.

You can enjoy this gluten-free treat all year long with whole wheat flour, egg whites, and unsweetened applesauce.

INGREDIENTS

- 1 cup of whole wheat flour
- 2 1/2 teaspoons of baking soda
- 1 teaspoon of ground ginger
- 1 teaspoon of ground allspice
- 1 teaspoon of ground cinnamon
- 1/2 cup of canola oil
- 2 egg whites
- 1 egg
- 2/3 cup of sugar
- 1 cup of molasses
- 1 cup of unsweetened applesauce
- 1 1/2 cup of all-purpose flour
- 1/2 teaspoon of salt
- 1 1/3 cup of reduced-fat frozen whipped topping, thawed

PREPARATIONS

- Preheat oven to 350 degrees F.
- Use paper liners to line muffin tins.
- Beat the egg whites, oil, egg and sugar until well blended in a large bowl.
- Add applesauce and molasses. Mix well.
- Combine flours, ginger, baking soda, cinnamon, allspice, and salt in a bowl.
- Beat in applesauce mixture gradually until blended.
- Spoon mixture into the muffin tins, filling each for about 2/3 full.
- Bake until a toothpick inserted in the center comes out clean, for about 18 to 22 minutes.
- Cool completely just before serving.
- Top each of the cupcake with 1 tablespoon of whipped topping.
- Serve and enjoy.

PREP TIME : 10 mins
COOK TIME : 22 mins
TOTAL TIME : 32 mins
YIELD : 24 cupcakes

BAKED CUSTARD

Do you know what I love about this recipe?

Baked Custard is so fantastic and easy to follow. You can add some nutmeg to the top before serving and top it with fresh, homemade whipped cream. Oh my goodness! So yummy!

You would want to make more and more of it even know though you didn't change anything in the recipe.

INGREDIENTS

- 1/4 teaspoon of ground nutmeg
- 1/4 teaspoon of ground cinnamon
- 3 teaspoons of vanilla extract
- 2-2/3 cups of whole milk
- 4 large eggs
- 2/3 cup of sugar
- 1/2 teaspoon of salt

PREPARATIONS

- Combine sugar, eggs, vanilla and spices in a bowl.
- Blend in milk and pour into a 1- and 1/2-quart baking dish.
- Place the baking dish inside a cake pan in the oven.
- Bake at 325 degrees until a knife inserted near the middle comes out clean, or for about an hour.
- Serve and enjoy.

PREP TIME : 10 mins
BAKE TIME : 6 mins
TOTAL TIME : 16 mins
YIELD : 6 servings

CHOCO MOUSSE

You won't imagine how good this will be until you give it a try!

This version of Chocolate Mousse is low carb and it will be so good. You can actually make a batch of it in a big bowl with the biggest serving spoon. It will be a knockout!

Is it Valentine's day already? Why not feel the love with this Chocolate Mousse using fancy glasses to serve? Smile!

INGREDIENTS

- 2 medium egg yolks
- 1/4 cup of granulated sugar substitute
- 1 teaspoon of pure vanilla extract
- 7 ounces (2 bars) of Perugina or Ghirardelli bittersweet or dark chocolate
- 2 tablespoons of strong coffee (you can use decaffeinated espresso)
- 2 tablespoons of orange liquor or Bourbon (optional)
- 3/4 cup plus 3 tablespoons of whipping cream
- 3 medium egg whites

PREPARATIONS

- Break up to 5 ounces of the chocolate.
- Place the chocolate, liquor and coffee in a small pot.
- In a larger pot of hot water that has been turned off the heat, cover and place the small pot and allow it to melt.
- Beat sugar substitute and egg yolks until frothy.
- Add the 3 tablespoons of whipping cream and vanilla into the egg mixture then beat to combine.
- Whisk the melted chocolate until shiny and smooth.
- Add the melted chocolate to the egg mixture slowly, stirring constantly.
- Beat egg whites until stiff peaks form.
- Fold in 1/4 of the egg whites into the chocolate to lighten the mixture.
- Fold in the rest of the egg whites.
- Grate about 2 ounces of chocolate on the medium side of a box grater. Fold into the mixture.
- Beat 3/4 cup of whipping cream until it holds its shape and triples in bulk.
- Fold the whipped cream into the rest of the mixture.
- Pour 6 glasses or into 1 large bowl.
- Chill for about 4 to 5 hours. Serve and enjoy.

PREP TIME : 25 mins
COOK TIME : 5 mins
TOTAL TIME : 30 mins
YIELD : 6 servings

CHRISTMAS COOKIES

These cookies could be easily shared and given to neighbors and friends. These cookies always lead to a baking bonanza to prepare for Christmas.

You should try icing these cookies when cold. And before baking, make sure you sprinkle with colored sugar. They would be perfect, fantastic and beautiful.

INGREDIENTS

- 2 teaspoons of baking powder
- 1/2 cup of skim milk
- 2 tablespoons of water
- 1 teaspoon of vanilla extract
- 1/2 cup of shortening
- 3 tablespoons of sugar substitute
- 1 egg
- Several drops of food coloring (optional)
- 2 1/2 cups of cake flour
- 1/2 teaspoon of salt

PREPARATIONS

- Cream the shortening.
- Add egg, sweetener and food coloring; beat well.
- Combine dry ingredients in a separate bowl; add the vanilla, milk and water.
- Put in the flour mixture and stir well.
- Chill the dough for about 2 to 4 hours.
- Preheat oven to 325 degrees F.
- Roll out 1/8 inch thick and cut the cookies into your desired shapes.
- Bake for about 8 to 10 minutes.
- Cool and store in an air-tight container.
- Enjoy.

PREP TIME : 10 mins
CHILL TIME : 4 hours
TOTAL TIME : 4 hours 10 mins
YIELD : 24 servings

ECLAIR BITES

While desserts from the bakery aren't always the best option if you're following a diabetic diet, that does not mean you will never get to enjoy your favorites again.

With this recipe for Eclair Bites, you can savor the sweetness of a classic bakery treat without going overboard.

I hope you enjoy it.

INGREDIENTS

- 1 1/2 stick margarine, melted
- 1 (4-serving size) package sugar-free instant French vanilla pudding mix
- 1 1/4 cup of low-fat milk
- 2 cups of reduced-fat graham cracker crumbs
- 1/2 cup of confectioners' sugar
- 2 cups of fat-free frozen whipped topping, thawed
- 3/4 cup of sugar-free chocolate frosting

PREPARATIONS

- Preheat oven to 350 degrees F.
- Use paper liners to line 18 mini muffin cups.
- Combine together sugar, graham crackers, and butter in a medium bowl; mix well.
- Press mixture evenly into paper liners.
- Press over the bottom and up sides of liners using your fingers.
- Bake until crust starts to brown or for about 5 minutes.
- Remove from the oven and leave to completely cool.
- Whisk pudding mixture and milk in a medium bowl.
- Fold in whipped topping.
- Place in a plastic bag and snip off one corner.
- Fill your graham cracker crusts evenly with pudding mixture.
- Heat frosting for about 10 to 15 seconds in a small microwave safe bowl.
- Stir until pourable and smooth.
- Place in a plastic bag and snip off one corner.
- Top pudding mixture with 1 dollop of chocolate frosting.
- Refrigerate until ready to serve, for about 4 hours.
- Serve and enjoy.

COOK TIME : 5 mins
CHILL TIME : 4 hours
TOTAL TIME : 4 hours 10 mins
YIELD : 18 servings

SNICKER DOODLES

Due to my taste, I added extra vanilla, and it felt good. You can add it too, if you truly want the full experience.

You'll be needing a little cinnamon on the rolling sugar to get that beautiful cinnamon coating. Snickerdoodles taste delicious and they are easy to make.

This might be your first-time making snickerdoodles, but I promise you that it's definitely going to work out great!

Enjoy.

- 1-1/2 cups of all-purpose flour
- 1/4 teaspoon of baking soda
- 1/4 teaspoon of cream of tartar
- 1 teaspoon of ground cinnamon
- 1/2 cup of softened butter
- 1 cup plus 2 tablespoons of sugar, divided
- 1 large egg, room temperature
- 1/2 teaspoon of vanilla extract

PREPARATIONS

- Preheat oven to 375 degrees F.
- Cream butter and 1 cup of sugar until fluffy and light.
- Beat in vanilla and egg.
- Whisk together baking soda, flour and cream of tartar in a separate bowl.
- Gradually beat into creamed mixture.
- Mix the rest of the sugar and cinnamon in small bowl.
- Shape dough into 1-inch balls.
- Roll in cinnamon sugar.
- Place 2-inches apart on ungreased baking sheets.
- Bake for about 10 to 12 minutes, until light browned.
- Remove from pans to wire racks to cool.
- Serve and enjoy.

PREP TIME : 20 mins
BAKE TIME : 10 mins
TOTAL TIME : 30 mins
YIELD : 2 and 1/2 dozen

LEMON BARS

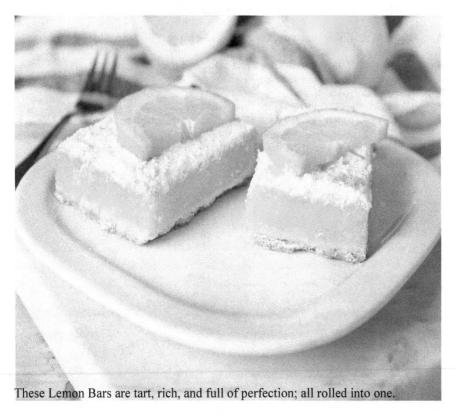

These Lemon Bars are tart, rich, and full of perfection; all rolled into one.

Put a smile on your friend's faces with this simple recipe today. The crust is the perfect thickness, and there is enough lemon custard in each bite to satisfy them.

This recipe makes a lot of crust and spreads into a 9 by 13 dish easily but makes a thinner bar. Make sure to increase the cooking time of the crust and fill an extra 5 to 10 minutes each if you'll be using a smaller baking dish, which is 8 by 11.

INGREDIENTS

- 4 eggs
- 1 and 1/2 cups of white sugar
- 1/4 cup of all-purpose flour
- 1 cup of butter, softened
- 1/2 cup of white sugar
- 2 cups of all-purpose flour
- 2 lemons, juiced

- Preheat oven to 350 degrees F.
- Blend together softened butter, 1/2 cup of sugar and 2 cups of flours in a medium bowl.
- Press into the bottom of an ungreased 9 by 13-inch pan.
- Bake in the preheated oven, for about 15 to 20 minutes, or until golden and firm.
- Whisk together the rest of the sugar and 1/4 cup of flour in a separate bowl.
- Whisk in the lemon juice and eggs.
- Pour over the baked crust.
- Bake for another 20 minutes in the preheated oven.
- The bars will firm up as they cool. Make another pan using limes instead of lemons for a festive tray, adding drops of green food coloring.
- After both pans have cooled, cut 2 into uniform 2-inch squares and arrange in a checkerboard fashion.
- Serve and enjoy.

PREP TIME : 15 mins
BAKE TIME : 40 mins
TOTAL TIME : 55 mins
YIELD : 36 servings

UPSIDE DOWN PINEAPPLE CAKE

This Classic Upside-Down Pineapple Cake boasts all the gooey, fruity, caramel-y goodness made for generations and generations to come - in addition to a secret shortcut so you can make it in a snap.

With your yellow cake mix, you can have this impressive dessert prepped for the oven within 15 minutes.

All you need to do is bake, flip, and bring to the table to add a colorful and sweet flourish to any party. Enjoy.

INGREDIENTS

- 1 can (20 ounces) of pineapple slices in juice, drained, juice reserved
- 1 jar (6 ounces) of maraschino cherries without stems, drained
- 1 box of yellow cake mix
- 1/4 cup of butter
- 1 cup of packed brown sugar
- Vegetable oil and eggs called for on cake mix box

PREPARATIONS

- Heat oven to 350 degrees F.
- Melt butter in the oven in 13 by 9-inch pan.
- Sprinkle brown sugar over butter.
- Arrange pineapples slices on brown sugar.
- In the center of each pineapple slice, place a cherry and arrange remaining cherries around slices; gently press into brown sugar.
- Add enough water into the reserved pineapple juice to measure 1 cup.
- Make your batter, substituting pineapple juice mixture for the water.
- Pour batter over cherries and pineapple.
- Bake for about 45 minutes or until toothpick inserted in center comes out clean.
- Loosen cake by running knife around side of the pan.
- Place your heatproof serving plate upside down onto a pan. turn the plate and pan over.
- Now, leave for just 5 minutes so the brown sugar topping can drizzle over cake.
- Remove pan and cool for about 30 minutes.
- Serve cool or warm.
- Enjoy.

PREP TIME : 15 mins
BAKE TIME : 1 hour 35 mins
TOTAL TIME : 1 hour 50 mins
YIELD : 12 servings

CARROT CAKE TOWERS

You don't have to be diabetic to enjoy this carrot cake. Carrot cake can be good or really, really bad, and this recipe has a flax-seed meal. But nothing could be further from the truth. This cake is super delicious and by adding the cream cheese, the frosting is divine.

These would be perfect for a party and it's a recipe you can make over and over again. They can be made into squares and triangles - it's your choice.

INGREDIENTS

- 1/4 teaspoon of salt
- 3 cups of finely shredded carrot about 6 medium-size (3 large for me)
- 1 cup of refrigerated or frozen egg product thawed, or 4 eggs, lightly beaten
- 1/2 cup of granulated sugar or sugar substitute blend-equivalent to 1/2 cup of granulated sugar
- 1/2 cup of packed brown sugar or brown sugar substitute blend-equivalent to 1/2 cup of brown sugar
- 1/2 cup of canola oil
- 1 1/2 cups of all-purpose flour
- 2/3 cup of flax seed meal
- 2 teaspoons of baking powder
- 1 teaspoon of pumpkin pie spice
- 1/2 teaspoon of baking soda
- 1 recipe of Fluffy Cream Cheese Frosting
- Coarsely shredded carrot optional

PREPARATIONS

- Preheat oven to 350 degrees F.
- Grease the bottom of a baking pan.
- Use waxed paper to line bottom of pan.
- Grease and flour the waxed paper and the sides of the pan lightly; set it aside.
- In a large bowl, stir together flax seed meal, flour, baking powder, baking soda, pumpkin pie spice, and salt; set it aside.
- In a separate large bowl, combine eggs, finely shredded carrot, brown sugar, granulated sugar and oil.
- Add egg mixture all at once into the flour mixture. Stir until well combined.
- Spoon batter into prepared pan, spreading evenly.
- Bake until a toothpick inserted near the center comes out clean, or for about 25 minutes.
- Cool cake in pan on a wire rack for about 10 minutes.
- Invert cake onto a wire rack and cool completely.
- Transfer cake onto a large cutting board.
- Make cutouts in the cake using a 2-inch round cutter, leaving as little space between the cutouts (you'd get 29 to 33 cutouts)
- For each of the servings, place one of the cake cutouts on a serving plate.
- Spread about 1 tablespoon of fluffy cream cheese frosting on top of the cake round.
- If desired, garnish with coarsely carrot, shredded.
- Serve and enjoy.

PREP TIME : 15 mins
BAKE TIME : 25 mins
TOTAL TIME : 50 mins
YIELD : 16 servings

GUMMY WORMS

This recipe makes dual-flavored raspberry and orange worms.

You can substitute other juices to change the flavors. You can as well make with a single flavor. Your kids would love it.

INGREDIENTS

- 12 tablespoons of sugar (separated)
- 8 tablespoons of corn syrup (separated)
- 2/3 cup of orange juice
- 8 tablespoons of unflavored gelatin (separated)
- 1/2 cup of cold water (divided)
- 2/3 cup of raspberry juice
- Optional: food coloring

PREPARATIONS

- Bring together all the ingredients.
- Prepare an 8 by 8-inch pan by using water to wet it.
- Place 4 tablespoons of gelatin inside a 1/4 cup of cold water to soften for about 5 minutes.
- Place the 6 tablespoons of sugar, raspberry juice, and 4 tablespoons of corn syrup in a medium saucepan over medium heat.
- Stir until sugar dissolves.
- Stir in the gelatin and continue until the gelatin dissolves.
- Now, add food coloring if you'll be using it.
- Pour into prepared pan and refrigerate until set, for about an hour.
- **Repeat procedure with orange juice by:**
- Placing 4 tablespoons of gelatin in 1/4 cup of cold water for about 5 minutes, to soften.
- Place the 6 tablespoons of sugar, raspberry juice, and 4 tablespoons of corn syrup in a medium saucepan over medium heat.
- Stir until sugar dissolves.
- Stir in the gelatin and continue until the gelatin dissolves.
- Now, add food coloring if you'll be using it.
- Remove from heat and allow it to cool in a pan for 10 minutes.
- Pour over raspberry layer and refrigerate until set, for an hour.
- Turn out of the pan when set and cut with a sharp knife into long, thin strips to resemble worms.
- Enjoy.

PREP TIME : 10 mins
COOL TIME : 20 mins
TOTAL TIME : 30 mins
YIELD : 8 servings

PUMPKIN PIE

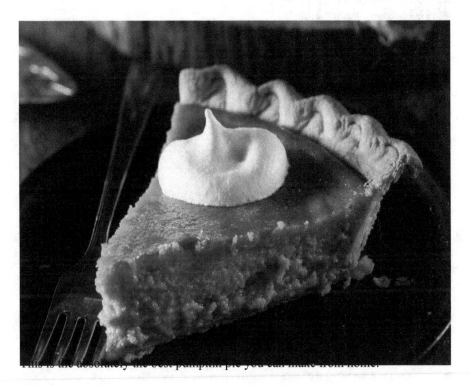

This is the absolutely the best pumpkin pie you can make from home.

Make it with fresh or canned pumpkin puree, and up to several days ahead.

I love this pie because they freeze well and it can be called the "Thanksgiving pie." But real Thanksgiving pie never looks so good and easy like that. I am in love with this recipe already. I hope you love it too.

INGREDIENTS

- 1/4 teaspoon of ground nutmeg
- 1/4 teaspoon of ground cloves
- 1/8 teaspoon of ground cardamom
- 1/2 teaspoon of lemon zest
- 2 cups of pumpkin pulp purée from a sugar pumpkin OR 1 15-ounce can of pumpkin purée (can also use puréed cooked butternut squash)
- 1 1/2 cup of heavy cream or one 12 ounces can of evaporated milk
- 2 large eggs plus the yolk of a third egg
- 1/2 cup of packed dark brown sugar
- 1/3 cup of white sugar
- 1/2 teaspoon of salt
- 2 teaspoons of cinnamon
- 1 teaspoon of ground ginger
- 1 good pie crust, chilled or frozen

PREPARATIONS

- Preheat your oven to 425 degrees F.
- In a large bowl, beat the eggs.
- Mix in the white sugar, brown sugar, cinnamon, salt, nutmeg, ground ginger, lemon zest, ground cloves and cardamom.
- Mix in the pumpkin puree.
- Stir in the cream and beat till everything is well combined.
- Pour the filling into a frozen pie shell.
- Bake at high temperature for 15 minutes at 425 degrees F.
- Lower the temperature to 350 degrees F after 15 minutes.
- Bake for about 45 to 55 minutes more.
- The pie is done when the knife inserted comes out clean.
- Cool the pumpkin pie on a wire rack for about 2 hours.
- Top with whipped cream
- Serve and enjoy.

PREP TIME : 20 mins
COOL TIME : 1 hour
TOTAL TIME : 1 hour 20 mins
YIELD : 8 servings

ALMOND MACAROONS

This recipe is the best for creating marvelous almond macaroons at home. The outsides are crisp and they are traditionally baked on edible rice paper; this is because they are extremely difficult to remove from the baking tray.

By the way, you can have some fun with fillings and flavors with these homemade almond macaroons. Enjoy.

INGREDIENTS

- 225 grams of ground almonds
- 200 grams of caster sugar, plus extra for sprinkling.
- 3 medium free-range egg whites.
- 15 whole blanched almonds split into half lengthways.

PREPARATIONS

- Mix the sugar and ground almonds into a large mixing bowl.
- Beat the egg whites with an electric mixer in a separate bowl on a slow speed until just frothy.
- Add the egg whites into the sugar and almonds, 1 tablespoon at a time, mixing after each spoonful.
- Keep going until the mixture is soft and not runny. You might need to use all the egg whites.
- Roll the mix into walnut size balls and space them apart on the baking trays.
- Flatten them slightly by pressing a blanched almond half into the top of each one.
- Sprinkle some caster sugar over the top of each, then leave them for about 10 to 15 minutes to sit.
- Heat the oven to 190 degrees C.
- Bake until pale golden brown, for about 15 to 20 minutes.
- Leave on the baking sheet for at least 10 minutes before transferring to a cooling rack to cool completely. They'll get harden as they cool.
- Serve with a cuppa.
- Enjoy.

PREP TIME : 20 mins
COOL TIME : 20 mins
TOTAL TIME : 40 mins
YIELD : 30 macaroons

CHOCO THICK COOKIES

These cookies are golden and beautiful on the outside, gooey and soft on the inside. It is loaded up with tons of melted chocolate.

The best thing about these cookies is their size. These cookies are hearty, thick, chewy, buttery, and extremely loaded with chocolate.

I hope you'll enjoy it.

INGREDIENTS

- 2 cups of all-purpose flour
- 1/2 teaspoon of salt
- 1/2 teaspoon of baking powder
- 3/4 cup of semi-sweet chocolate chips
- 1/4 cup of chopped pecans
- 1/2 cup of unsalted butter, room temperature
- 3/4 cup of light brown sugar
- 1/4 cup of white sugar
- 1 large egg
- 1 teaspoon of vanilla extract

PREPARATIONS

- Use a silicone baking mat to line a large baking sheet; set it aside.
- Add the sugars and butter in a large mixing bowl.
- Cream the butter and sugars using a stand mixer or a hand together until fluffy.
- Add in the vanilla, large egg, then mix until combined.
- Add the baking powder, flour, and salt.
- Mix until well combined. The dough might seem to be crumbling.
- Pour in the pecans and chocolate chips and mix them using your hands.
- Divide the dough into 6 pieces.
- Gently form into a cookie shape and place on the baking sheet.
- Bake the cookies until golden brown, or for about 18 minutes.
- Let the cookies cool on the baking sheet for at 5 minutes, then remove to a wire rack to continue cooling.
- Serve and enjoy.

PREP TIME : 10 mins
COOK TIME : 16 mins
CHILL TIME : 30 mins
TOTAL TIME : 56 mins
YIELD : 6 servings

POACHED PEARS

Your Poached Pears can be served with some mascarpone cheese, a scoop of vanilla ice cream, or whipped cream for an impressive diabetic dessert.

It's an easy and simple recipe that is absolutely elegant. They have a great balance of spice, sweet and fruity flavors.

It's mildly sweet and crisp making them the perfect canvas for all the flavors in the poaching liquid.

INGREDIENTS

- 1 teaspoon of ground nutmeg
- 4 whole pears
- 1/2 cup of fresh raspberries
- 1 cup of orange juice
- 1/4 cup of apple juice
- 1 teaspoon of ground cinnamon
- 2 tablespoons of orange zest

PREPARATIONS

- Mix together apple juice, orange juice, nutmeg, and ground cinnamon in a small bowl.
- Stir ingredients until well mixed; set it aside.
- Peel the pears and leave the stems.
- Remove the core from the bottom of the pear and in a shallow saucepan, place the pears.
- Pour over juice mixture into the pan and set over medium heat.
- Simmer your pears for about 30 minutes, turning frequently.
- Don't bring liquid to a boil.
- Transfer the pears to individual plates.
- Garnish with orange zest and raspberries.
- Serve immediately and enjoy.

PREP TIME : 10 mins
COOK TIME : 30 mins
TOTAL TIME : 40 mins
YIELD : 4 servings

PUMPKIN MOUSSE

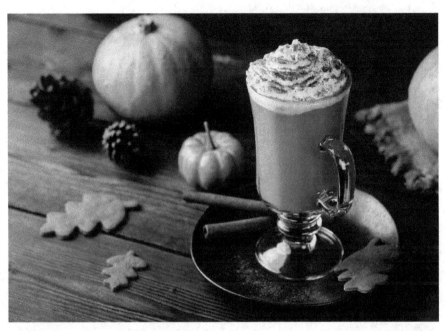

Pumpkin mousse is fluffy, creamy, melt in your mouth perfection, and it is one of my family's favorite pumpkin desserts.

When I make it every year, another die-heard pumpkin-hater falls prey to its awesomeness. You need to give it a try!

INGREDIENTS

- 2 tablespoons of maple syrup
- 1/2 teaspoon of pure vanilla extract
- 1 cup of whole milk
- 1 1/2 cup of heavy cream
- 1 (3.4 ounces) package of instant vanilla pudding
- 1 teaspoon of pumpkin spice
- 1/2 teaspoon of cinnamon, plus more for garnish
- 1/2 teaspoon of kosher salt
- 1 (15-ounces) can of pumpkin purée

PREPARATIONS

- Whisk together spices, pudding mix and salt in a large bowl.
- Add maple syrup, vanilla, pumpkin, and whole milk, then beat until smooth with a hand mixer.
- Whip heavy cream for about 3 to 4 minutes, until stiff peaks form in another large bowl.
- Fold 2/3 of the whipped cream into the pumpkin mixture until smooth.
- Spoon into serving dishes.
- Top with the remaining whipped cream.
- Garnish with a sprinkle of cinnamon.
- Serve and enjoy.

PREP TIME : 10 mins
COOK TIME : 0 mins
TOTAL TIME : 10 mins
YIELD : 4 servings

YOGURT BLUEBERRY POPSICLES

Yogurt Blueberry Popsicles are made with protein-packed three (3) ingredients that are so healthy for the body.

These popsicles hit the spot when the weather heats up. It's a diabetic and gluten-free treat you need to try today.

INGREDIENTS

- 2 cups of blueberries
- 2 tablespoons of honey or agave
- 2 cups of vanilla Greek yogurt or any flavor of your choice

PREPARATIONS

- In a food processor or blender, blend the blueberries on high speed until nearly liquified into a smoothie.
- In a large bowl, pour the thick blueberry liquid.
- Stir in the honey/agave.
- Add the yogurt and gently mix everything together.
- For a swirly look for your popsicles - do not fully blend the blueberries and yogurt.
- The mixture will be thick. Now, taste it and if you want it sweeter, you can add a little more honey/agave.
- Pour the mixture evenly into each of the popsicle molds.
- You can insert them before freezing if your popsicle mold has slots for sticks. If not, freeze for about 2 hours.
- Put a wooden popsicle stick in the middle.
- Continue to freeze for an additional 5 hours or over the night.
- Run the popsicle molds under warm water to remove easily.
- Eat on a hot day.
- Serve and enjoy.

PREP TIME : 10 mins
COOK TIME : 0 mins
TOTAL TIME : 6 to 8 hours
YIELD : 6 popsicles

LEMON PIE CURD

Lemon Pie Curd is a delicious dessert packed with coconut flour pie crust and sugar-free lemon curd. It's 100% paleo, keto, and gluten-free.

This recipe is perfect when served with sugar-free meringue and strawberries. I have tested this recipe before and I love it so much. You should add it to your favorites - so healthy.

INGREDIENTS

- 1 coconut flour pie crust
- Sugar Free Lemon Pie Curd
- 2 Egg Yolk - keep egg white for meringue
- 1/2 cup of Butter or coconut oil, melted
- 1/2 cup of Lemon Juice or juice of about 5 small lemons
- 2 Eggs
- 1/4 cup of Erythritol - erythritol or monk fruit sugar
- Sugar Free Meringue Frosting
- 2 egg whites
- 1/4 cup of Erythritol

PREPARATIONS

- Prepare your Coconut Flour Pie Crust
  Preparing the Lemon Pie Curd:
- In a saucepan, whisk the lemon juice, eggs, sweetener, and egg yolks together.
- Bring to a medium heat and add the butter or coconut oil, stirring continuously to prevent the eggs from scrambling and cooking.
- Increase the heat to medium high when the coconut oil is melted, keep stirring until it thickens up.
- Remove from heat and transfer into a bowl to cool down at room temperature for about 15 minutes.
- Fill in the coconut flour pie crust with the lemon pie curd.
- Refrigerate the lemon pie to firm up for at least 2 hours.
  Preparing the Meringue Frosting:
- Add the meringue before serving.
- Whisk the egg whites in a bowl until it starts producing a good volume.
- This is usually 30 seconds on high speed.
- Keep whisking on high speed and add the sugar free crystal sweetener of your choice slowly.
- After 1 minute, the meringue should be really fluffy and triple its volume.
- Tip the bowl upside down to check if the meringue is ready.
- Transfer on the top of the lemon pie curd if it sticks to the bowl.
- Torch the top of the meringue or place for 2 minutes in the oven or grill more until the top is brown slightly.
- Serve and enjoy.

PREP TIME : 20 mins
COOK TIME : 20 mins
TOTAL TIME : 40 mins
YIELD : 8 servings

BOUNTY BARS

Bounty bars are healthy, raw homemade candy bars that are 100% keto, paleo, sugar-free, and diabetic friendly.

This recipe can be made within 30 minutes, with only four ingredients. The bars are mainly made of healthy fats from coconut oil. These bars do not contain many calories and they are very filling.

You can adjust the sweetness with extra stevia drops if you have a really sweet tooth.

INGREDIENTS

- 2 cups of unsweetened desiccated coconut
- 1/3 cup of Coconut oil, melted, at room temperature
- Half cup of Canned Coconut cream, shake the can before use, full-fat minimum 30% fat, at room temperature (not cold)
- 1/3 cup of Erythritol
Chocolate Coating:
- 6 ounces of Sugar-free Chocolate Chips
- 2 teaspoon of Coconut oil
- 1-2 Monk Fruit Drops or Stevia Drops

PREPARATIONS

- Cover a square 9 by 9 inch pan with parchment paper and set it aside.
- Add melted coconut oil, erythritol, desiccated coconut and canned coconut cream in a food processor.
- Process on high speed, for at least 1 minute.
- You may have to process for 20 seconds. Stop and scrape down the bowl and repeat until it comes together into a fine wet coconut batter.
- Press the raw dough onto the prepared pan.
- Make sure there's no air left between the batter.
- Use your hands to press the batter and use spatula to flatten the surface.
- Freeze for 10 minutes to firm up.
- Don't freeze them too long or they might get so much hard as it's difficult to cut them into bars - they might break into pieces.
- But they will still look delicious and less pretty.
- Remove from the freezer.
- Lift up the parchment paper to release the coconut block from the pan.
- Place on a chopping board.
- Cut into 20 rectangles using a sharp knife.
- Shape each rectangle into your hands to form round borders like the real Bounty Bar if you want.
- Place each formed bounty bars on plate covered with parchment paper.
- Set it aside in the freezer while you prepare the chocolate coating.
- Meanwhile, in the microwave, melt the sugar free chocolate chips with coconut oil.
- Microwave until fully melted by 30 seconds.
- Add stevia drops to adjust sweetness to your taste if you want.
- Dip each coconut bar into the melted chocolate mixture using 2 forks.
- Freeze again to set the chocolate shell when all the bars have been covered with chocolate.
- Store the bounty bars in the fridge in an airtight container for up to a month or freeze.
- Defrost for about half hour before eating.
- Serve and enjoy.

PREP TIME : 10 mins
COOK TIME : 0 mins
TOTAL TIME : 30 mins
YIELD : 20 bars

COTTAGE CHEESE

What I love about Cottage Cheese is the flavor. It always makes my day. This recipe is a must-have at any family potluck, church, dinner, or holiday gatherings. You can pretty much use any Jell-o you prefer. It's just as good with just about any.

You can also add chopped pecans for texture if you want.

Enjoy!

EASY DIABETIC DESSERT RECIPES

INGREDIENTS

- 3 cups of low-fat cottage cheese
- 2 (0.3 ounces) packages of sugar-free lemon-flavored Jell-O mix
- 1 (8 ounces) container of lite frozen whipped topping, thawed

PREPARATIONS

- In a food processor, place the cottage cheese and blend until creamy.
- Whisk in the flavored gelatin powder.
- Fold in the thawed whipped topping.
- Refrigerate until serving.
- Serve and enjoy.

PREP TIME : 5 mins
ADDITIONAL TIME : 30 mins
TOTAL TIME : 35 mins
YIELD : 6 servings

BERRY COBBLER

This classic dessert has zero sugar added so all the sweetness comes from the berries themselves. *Smile* - you would love them!

You can choose your favorite berries to put into this berry cobbler recipe. It's up to you.

Filling:
- 3 tablespoons of cornstarch
- 4 cups of blackberries or marionberries, boysenberries, blueberries
- 1 packet of sweetener up to 2 packets, as sweet as 2 teaspoons of sugar each, optional
- 3 tablespoons of water
- 1/2 cup of fruit-sweet boysenberry syrup or blueberry syrup
- 3/4 teaspoon of cinnamon

Dough:
- 1 cup of unbleached flour
- 2 tablespoons of apple juice concentrate
- 1/4 cup of low-fat fruit-sweet berry yogurt or cherry flavor
- 1 and 1/2 teaspoon of baking powder
- 1/2 teaspoon of salt
- 2 tablespoons of butter, melted

- Preheat the oven to 400 degrees F.
- Use nonstick spray to cover a deep-dish pie pan.

Making the filling:
- Stir cornstarch into the water until dissolved.
- Mix in cinnamon and syrup.
- Let it sit and set it aside.

Making the dough:
- Sift together baking powder, flour and salt.
- Combine juice concentrate, butter and yogurt in a separate bowl.
- Pour wet ingredients over the dry ingredients.
- Gently blend with a fork for about 20 to 30 seconds.
- Knead the dough for about 20 to 30 more seconds.
- Press dough into approximately 1/4 to 1/2 inch thickness on a floured surface and wide enough to cover your pan.

Making the pie:
- Fold rinsed, drained berries into filling mixture.
- Pour berry filling into a greased pan.
- Over the top, set the cobbler dough, making the dough surface as even as possible.
- Press the dough against the sides of the pan.
- Cut a design in the dough for air ventilation.
- Turn oven down to 375 degrees F.
- Bake until the dough is light brown, or for about 20 to 25 minutes.
- Let it cool and serve.
- Enjoy.

PREP TIME : 15 mins
COOK TIME : 25 mins
TOTAL TIME : 40 mins
YIELD : 8 servings

CHOCO BANANA BITES

Choco Banana Bites are super easy to make and always a hit with everyone. They are so delicious - they taste like a treat!

And they are made with wholesome ingredients; they are refreshing, convenient, and very easy to make. You just need to grab a bite from the freezer whenever you need it and it's pretty hot on the outside.

You would love it!

INGREDIENTS

- 3 small (about 6-inches long) ripe bananas, each cut into 6 (1-inch.) slices
- 18 cocktail picks
- 2 tablespoons of unsweetened shredded dried coconut, toasted
- 2 tablespoons of chopped toasted almonds
- 1/2 teaspoon of sea salt flakes (such as Maldon)
- 5 ounces (85% cacao) of dark chocolate, finely chopped
- 2 teaspoons of coconut oil

PREPARATIONS

- Skewer each banana slice with 1 cocktail pick and place it on a parchment lined baking sheet.
- Freeze for an hour.
- Pour water into a depth of 1-inch bottom of a double boiler and set over medium heat; bring to a boil.
- Reduce heat to medium-low, then simmer.
- Place oil and chocolate in top of the double boiler and cook, turning often, until mixture is smooth and chocolate melts, or for about 4 minutes.
- In the chocolate mixture, dip 1 skewered banana slice.
- Sprinkle immediately with a pinch of coconut and return to a baking sheet.
- Repeat procedure with the rest of the coconut for 5 extra banana slices and almonds for 6 banana slices.
- Then with the sea salt for the remaining 6 banana slices.
- Freeze bites before serving, or for about an hour.
- Serve and enjoy.

PREP TIME : 12 mins
COOK TIME : 0 mins
TOTAL TIME : 2 hour 12 mins
YIELD : 18 bites

FIG ORANGE PIE

Fig orange pies are perfect for brunch gatherings, a sweet treat with your afternoon tea, and a diabetic-friendly dessert.

You just have to pick up one of these fruit-filled pastries and bite in. You would fall in love with this; it's pretty satisfying.

Enjoy!

INGREDIENTS

- 1 cup all-purpose flour
- 3 fresh figs or 8 dried Mission figs
- 1 medium orange
- 1/4 cup of low-sugar orange marmalade
- Fat-free milk
- 1 teaspoon of powdered sugar
- 1/4 cup white whole-wheat flour or whole-wheat flour
- 2 tablespoons flax-seed meal
- 1/4 teaspoon salt
- 1/3 cup 60% to 70% tub-style vegetable oil spread, chilled
- 3-4 tablespoons cold water, divided

PREPARATIONS

- Preheat oven to 400 degrees F.
- Use parchment paper to line a large baking sheet; set it aside.
- Stir together flax-seeds meal, flours and salt in a medium bowl.
- Cut in chilled vegetable oil spread until pieces are pea size using a pastry blender.
- Sprinkle 1 tablespoon of cold water over part of the flour mixture. toss with a fork gently.
- Push moistened dough to the side of the bowl.
- Repeat moistening the flour mixture using 1 tablespoon of cold water at a time, until all the flour mixture is moistened.
- Divide the dough into 8 equal portions.
- Remove stems from figs.
- Place dried figs in a small bowl with enough boiling water to cover if you'll be using dried figs; let it stand for about 5 minutes to rehydrate, and then drain well.
- Chop the fresh or rehydrated dried figs.
- Shred enough orange peel to make 1/4 teaspoon and set it aside.
- Peel and chop the sections.
- Combine the chopped orange, figs, marmalade, and the shredded orange peel in a medium bowl. Stir well until combined.
- Roll each portion of the pastry dough on a lightly floured surface into 4-inch circle.
- Spoon the fig mixture atop the dough circles.
- Spread to an even layer, leave a 3/4-inch border on the edges.
- Moisten the edges of the dough circles using a little water.
- Fold the dough circles in half to make semi-circles.
- Press the edges to seal using the tines of a fork.
- Place the pies 2-inches apart on the prepared baking sheet.
- Make small slashes on the top of the pies to allow the steam to escape.
- Brush with milk lightly.
- Bake until the tops are golden brown, or for about 17 to 20 minutes.
- Transfer onto a wire rack. Cool for about 15 minutes.
- Sprinkle with powdered sugar lightly.
- Serve and enjoy.

PREP TIME : 40 mins
ADDITIONAL TIME : 0 mins
TOTAL TIME : 1 hour

YIELD : 8 servings

MICROWAVE POPCORN

What I love about this Microwave Popcorn is that it's perfect for when it's chilly outside. It's packed with cocoa. If you are a fan of cocoa, you should have an interest in trying this recipe.

Enjoy the best two spectacular snacks with this delicately sweetened popcorn treat made inside the microwave.

Enjoy.

INGREDIENTS

- 1/2 teaspoon of cocoa powder
- 1/2 teaspoon of sugar
- Pinch of salt
- 1 and 1/2 tablespoons of popcorn kernels
- 1/2 teaspoon of coconut oil

PREPARATIONS

- Add popcorn kernels to a brown paper bag.
- Fold the top of the bag over 3 times.
- Microwave for about 1 and half minutes, or until the popping stops.
- In a small microwave-safe bowl, place coconut oil and microwave for about 20 seconds, until melted. Stir with a fork.
- Add the cocoa powder, oil, salt, and sugar to the bag over the popped popcorn.
- Fold the top of the bag.
- Hold closed and shake to coat.
- Serve and enjoy.

PREP TIME : 5 mins
ADDITIONAL TIME : 0 mins
TOTAL TIME : 5 mins
YIELD : 1 serving

BLOSSOM COOKIES WITH PEANUT BUTTER

These Blossom Peanut Butter Cookies are delicious on their own—a healthier take on the best Christmas cookies around.

You can make them better by pressing a piece of dark chocolate candy into each of the hot cookies immediately after the cookies come out of the oven.

So yummy!

INGREDIENTS

- 1 cup of all-purpose flour
- 1/3 cup of whole-wheat flour
- 1/2 teaspoon of baking powder
- 1/2 teaspoon of baking soda
- 1/4 teaspoon of salt
- 1 cup of packed light brown sugar
- 1/4 cup of natural peanut butter
- 2 tablespoons of canola oil
- 1 large egg
- 1 teaspoon of vanilla extract
- 1 tablespoon of water
- 28 large dark chocolate candy pieces, unwrapped

PREPARATIONS

- Preheat oven to 350 degrees F.
- Use cooking spray to coat 2 baking sheets.
- Combine peanut butter, brown sugar, egg, oil and vanilla in a mixing bowl.
- Add water and beat until smooth with an electric mixer.
- Stir together whole-wheat flours and all-purpose, baking soda and salt in a small bowl.
- Stir the dry ingredients into the brown sugar mixture until well combined.
- Roll the dough between your palms into balls using wet hands and 1 tablespoon for each.
- Flatten each ball into half-inch thick dish.
- Place 2 inches apart on the prepared baking sheets.
- Bake the cookies, one sheet at a time for about 8 to 9 minutes, until golden.
- Press a chocolate piece immediately into each cookie's center.
- Transfer onto a wire rack to cool. Serve and enjoy.

PREP TIME : 30 mins
ADDITIONAL TIME : 0 mins
TOTAL TIME : 1 hour
YIELD : 28 servings

APPLE NUT WEDGES

Apple Nut Wedges can be served warm with a dollop of a yogurt blend topping.

You can use MacIntosh apples for softer apple chunks. It's easy to prepare, diabetic-friendly, and it's super-duper delicious!

Enjoy!

- 1/8 teaspoon of salt
- 2 large apples, cored and chopped (2 cups)
- 1/2 cup of chopped walnuts or pecans, toasted
- 1/2 cup of light sour cream
- 1/4 cup of vanilla low-fat yogurt sweetened with artificial sweetener
- 1/2 teaspoon of vanilla
- Nonstick cooking spray
- 1 egg
- 2 egg whites
- 2/3 cup of packed brown sugar or brown sugar substitute blend equivalent to 2/3 cup of brown sugar
- 1 teaspoon of vanilla
- 1/3 cup of all-purpose flour
- 3/4 teaspoon of baking soda

PREPARATIONS

- Preheat oven to 325 degrees F.
- Use cooking spray to coat a 9-inch pie plate and set it aside.
- Combine egg whites, egg, brown sugar, and 1 teaspoon of vanilla in a large bowl.
- Beat with an electric mixer on medium speed until smooth, or for about 1 minute.
- Stir together baking soda, flour, and salt in a small bowl.
- Add flour mixture into the egg mixture. Stir until well combined.
- Fold in nuts and apples and spread batter evenly in the prepared pie plate.
- Bake until center is set, or for about 25 to 30 minutes.
- Slightly cool on a wire rack.
- For topping: whisk together yogurt, sour cream and 1/2 teaspoon of vanilla in a small bowl.
- To serve, cut dessert into wedges.
- Serve warm and enjoy.

PREP TIME : 25 mins
ADDITIONAL TIME : 0 mins
TOTAL TIME : 50 mins
YIELD : 8 servings

COCOA FUDGE COOKIES

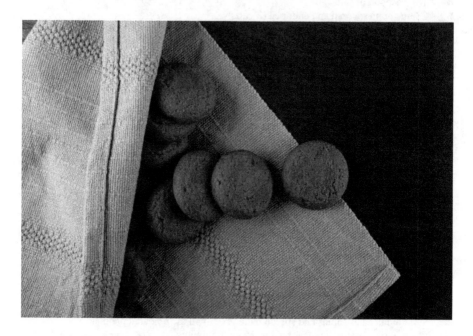

Cocoa Fudge Cookies is a dessert you can prepare in the saucepan. They are incredibly easy and freshly baked as well.

These cookies have crisp edges and chewy centers - so yummy.

You can make them with natural unsweetened cocoa powder or Dutch processed. I hope you love it, it would be great if you could give me feedback on them when you prepare it.

INGREDIENTS

- 7 tablespoons of unsweetened cocoa
- 2/3 cup of granulated sugar
- 1/3 cup of packed brown sugar
- 1/3 cup of plain low-fat yogurt
- 1 cup of all-purpose flour
- 1/4 teaspoon of baking soda
- 1/8 teaspoon of salt
- 5 tablespoons of butter
- 1 teaspoon of vanilla extract cooking spray

PREPARATIONS

- Preheat oven to 350 degrees F.
- Spoon flour into a dry measuring cup.
- Level using a knife.
- Combine soda, flour, and salt; set it aside.
- In a large saucepan, melt butter over a medium heat.
- Remove from the heat; stir in sugars and cocoa powder.
- Add vanilla and yogurt, stir to combine.
- Add flour mixture, stir until moist.
- Drop level tablespoons 2 inches apart onto baking sheets coat with cooking spray.
- Bake at 350 degrees until almost set, or for about 8 to 10 minutes.
- Cool on pans until firm, or for about 2 to 3 minutes.
- Remove cookies from pans, cool on wire racks.
- Serve and enjoy.

PREP TIME : 20 mins
ADDITIONAL TIME : 0 mins
TOTAL TIME : 40 mins
YIELD : 2 dozen

THUMBPRINT COOKIES WITH RASPBERRY

Adding some colors to your cookie tray with these jam-filled thumbprints will be so amazing. This recipe could be your healthy alternative for the next holiday, church gathering, or school party.

To save time, you can use pre-made raspberry jam to save time and they would be a hit. You need to add this to your favorites.

I hope you love it. Enjoy!

- 5 tablespoons butter, softened 1/4 teaspoon vanilla extract
- 1 large egg white
- 3/4 cup (3 ounces) grated almond paste 2/3 cup sugar
- 1 1/4 cups all-purpose flour (about 5 1/2 ounces) 1/4 teaspoon salt
- 6 tablespoons Raspberry Refrigerator Jam

PREPARATIONS

- Preheat the oven to 325 degrees F.
- Use parchment paper to line 2 large baking sheets, secure to baking sheet with masking top.
- In a bowl, place almond pasta, sugar and butter in a bowl.
- Beat with mixture at a medium speed until light and fluffy, or for about 4 minutes.
- Spoon flour into dry measuring cups and level using your knife.
- Add salt and flour until well combined and until golden.
- Remove cakes from the pans and cool on wire racks.
- Spoon about 1/2 teaspoon raspberry refrigerator jam in the center of each of the cookie.

Notes:

- Almond paste makes the dough pliable and moist.
- Look for it in the supermarket baking aisle.
- The large holes of box grater work well for grating the almond paste.
- To make deeper indentations in the cookies, use a wine cork.
- Bake both pans of the cookies at the same time.
- Rotate the pans in the oven halfway through baking time for even browning.
- Serve and enjoy.

PREP TIME : 20 mins
ADDITIONAL TIME : 0 mins
TOTAL TIME : 40 mins
YIELD : 2 dozen

SUGAR FREE BUCKEYE BALLS

These delicious tasting Sugar Free Buckeye Balls are the perfect treat to share with your families and friends. They are low in carbs and diabetic-friendly because they're made with zero sugar.

We'll be adding sugar free peanut butter to this recipe. They actually work together in creating delicious taste.

INGREDIENTS

- 6 cups of Sugar Free Powdered Sugar
- 1 teaspoon of Vanilla Extract
- 1 1/2 cups of Sugar Free Peanut Butter
- 1 cup of Butter very soft
- 4 cups of Sugar Free Chocolate Chips

PREPARATIONS

- Prepare a baking sheet with wax paper. Set it aside.
- Cream together the sugar-free peanut butter, vanilla extract and sugar free powdered sugar in a mixing bowl.
- Form the mixture into 1 - 1 1/2-inches balls by rolling the dough in your hands.
- Place each of the ball on the wax prepared baking sheet.
- Place the prepared balls into the freezer for about 25 minutes, or until hard.
- Melt the chocolate in a microwave when you're ready to dip the balls in the chocolate or use the double boiler method.
- Stir the chocolate melts in well.
- Remove the peanut butter balls from the freezer and dip each of them into the chocolate. You can leave the area around where you can put your toothpick.
- Then place each ball back to the wax paper and refrigerate them.
- Melt more if you run low on chocolate.
- Serve and enjoy.

NOTE:
The buckeye balls should be stored in an airtight container in the refrigerator to keep them nice and fresh. Stored in this way they will keep for about 1 month. You can also freeze buckeyes in an airtight container or freezer Ziploc bag for up to 3 months.

PREP TIME : 20 mins
FREEZING TIME : 35 mins
TOTAL TIME : 55 mins
YIELD : 36 balls

BAKED APPLE CRISP

Are you wondering if you can bake this dessert on your grill?

Yes, you can. This is a traditional apple crisp that is baked directly on the grill. When you taste this recipe for the first time, you will be moved to add it to your favorite. It's so fantastic and a great addition to your Thanksgiving dinner.

It's yummy!

INGREDIENTS

- 2 teaspoons of ground cinnamon
- 2 teaspoons of baking powder
- 3/4 teaspoon of salt
- 1/2 cup (4 ounces) of butter
- 10 apples (about 5 pounds), preferably a mixture of Granny Smith and Golden Delicious
- 2 cups of all-purpose flour
- 1 cup of sugar
- 2 large eggs
- Vanilla ice cream (optional)

PREPARATIONS

- Melt butter over a low heat and set it aside.
- Peel, core and cut apples into 1/3-inch-thick slices.
- In a 9 by 13-inch baking pan, place apples and spread to be level.
- Mix flour, cinnamon, sugar, salt and baking powder in a bowl.
- Drop in eggs and mix with a fork or pastry blender until crumbly.
- Spread toppings evenly over apples.
- Drizzle with the melted butter.
- Prepare your grill for indirect heat at 350 degrees to 400 degrees F.
- On the grill, place the apple crisp and cover with barbecue.
- Cook until the apples are bubbling and the topping is browned, or for about 40 to 45 minutes.
- Serve warm with vanilla ice cream as an optional extra.
- **Apple Crisp:** Smoke this apple crisp if you really love the flavor of smoke.
- Cover 1/3 cup of apple-wood chips with water, then soak for 30 minutes and drain.
- Scatter the chips over the coals just before you place the apple crisp on the grate.
- Serve and enjoy.

PREP TIME : 10 mins
COOK TIME : 65 mins
TOTAL TIME : 85 mins
YIELD : 8 to 10 servings

CHEESE PITTAS

Cheese Pittas is one of my favorites. You can dump them into your favorite soup or have them together on their own for an easy and quick lunch that's always a hit.

With just six ingredients, your grilled cheese pitas can be ready-to-eat.

Cheese Pittas benefit from the absorbing, compressing, union-promoting nature of the astringent taste.

INGREDIENTS

- 1-2 teaspoon of butter or as needed
- 2 fluffy pittas or naan flat bread
- 4 slices of ripe tomato
- 2 handfuls baby spinach
- 4 ounces of grated cheese (you can use mozzarella with Havarti)
- salt and pepper to taste

PREPARATIONS

- Prep your cheese and veggies so they are ready to go.
- Heat a pan to medium high heat.
- Add 1 teaspoon of butter.
- Add a pitta to the pan once the butter begins to bubble.
- Top with spinach, cheese and tomato with a little extra cheese on the top.
- Top with the remaining pitta round.
- Now, grill.
- For an extra melty and hot center, pop a clear pot lid on top.
- Add another teaspoon of butter to the pan before flipping or you can feel free to spread it on top of the dry side of the pitta.
- If you're using one, pop your lid back and grill each side, or until it turns golden brown with a melty center.
- Cut into 4 wedges.
- Serve and enjoy.

PREP TIME : 5 mins
COOK TIME : 8 mins
TOTAL TIME : 13 mins
YIELD : 2 servings

FRUIT KABOBS

Do you know that grilling fruit caramelizes the natural sugars in them for a comfortable, sweet, and healthy dessert? It would be great if you try this grilled fruit kabobs this summer.

The natural sugars in the fruit will caramelize over the heat and bring out the fruit's sweet flavor. You'll realize that this recipe is a healthy and delicious dessert that tastes great. It not only just takes a couple of minutes on the grill, but it's so easy to prepare.

Serve it with a scoop of ice cream or some yogurt. You would love it!

INGREDIENTS

- 1 cup of cantaloupe chunks cut into 1-inch pieces
- 1 cup of strawberries stems removed
- 1 cup of pineapple chunks cut into 1-inch pieces
- 1 banana cut 1-inch pieces
- Coconut oil spray
- 1 tablespoon of maple syrup for drizzling
- Vanilla yogurt for dipping (optional)

PREPARATIONS

- Inside water, soak the skewers for about 20 minutes to prevent the skewers from burning while grilling them.

Making the fruit kabobs:
- Thread 2 pieces each of pineapple, banana, cantaloupe and strawberry onto a skewer.
- Repeat this process to assemble as many skewers as you'd like to prepare.
- Drizzle with maple syrup and olive oil.
- Grill on a preheated grill until the fruit chars and softens, turning occasionally for about 10 minutes.
- Enjoy immediately.
- Dip in yogurt as an optional extra.

PREP TIME : 10 mins
COOK TIME : 2 mins
TOTAL TIME : 12 mins
YIELD : 6 servings

If you enjoyed this book, please let me know your thoughts by leaving a short review on **Amazon**

THANK

YOU.

5 Easy Diabetic Dessert Recipes

Stella - Waters

CPSIA information can be obtained
at www.ICGtesting.com
Printed in the USA
LVHW050549231220
674889LV00009B/402